Guide to Aromatherapy

ALTERNATIVE THERAPIES

D0019272

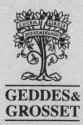

GEDDES & GROSSET

CAUTION

Do not undertake any course of treatment without the advice of your doctor. Never stop taking medication without the agreement of your doctor.

Some essential oils, when used inappropriately, can prove to be highly toxic. Some essential oils are unsuitable for use at home. Consult a professional aromatherapist before undertaking any treatment with essential oils.

Do not use essential oils in pregnancy, or on babies and young children, without the advice of a trained aromatherapist.

Some medical conditions contra-indicate the use of certain essential oils and/or massage.

Do not ingest essential oils. Do not use essential oils in the eyes.

Do not use essential oils undiluted on the skin unless otherwise indicated.

If using homeopathy or herbal medicine, seek the advice of the relevant practitioner as well as that of an aromatherapist.

© 1999 Geddes & Grosset,
David Dale House, New Lanark, ML11 9DJ, Scotland

First published 1999, reprinted 1999, 2007

Cover photograph courtesy of EyeWire

ISBN 978 1 85534 689 5

Printed and bound in India

Contents

What is Aromatherapy?

Aromatherapy is the term used for a form of therapy that makes use of the essential oils of a large number of aromatic plants, shrubs and trees. The oils extracted from the plants can be used in a variety of different ways, for the treatment of both medical and psychological conditions, for cosmetic purposes, or simply for pleasure. Essential oils can affect both the physical and mental state of an individual, and scientific research continues into the precise manner in which the oils take effect.

Aromatherapy has been practised for a very long time. Its rise in popularity in recent years has partially contributed to its being labelled by some people as a New Age therapy, but this is hardly an appropriate way to describe a use of plants and essential oils that has a history of several hundreds of years. Moreover, it is unfortunate that the New Age label brings with it more than a little prejudice. New Age is a term that sceptics tend to use in a derogatory sense, as if New Age equates with 'mumbo-jumbo'. What the sceptics will be unlikely to admit is that they, like all of us, probably indulge in some sort of aromatherapy in their everyday lives, whether they realise it or not.

Qualified aromatherapists require a great deal of knowledge and expertise to enable them to practise. Their skills can be invaluable in the treatment of many ailments, whether these ailments require additional conventional medical treatment or not. Sometimes aromatherapy will be used as a treatment. It has many applications in the treatment of a wide variety of ailments, some relatively minor, others of a more serious nature. As research into the subject continues, so the possibilities of aromatherapy expand. At other times, aromatherapy will be used as a palliative. Where it is used properly, it can do much to make a person feel better in himself or herself, even if it cannot effect a cure.

We are often our own aromatherapists in a sense. Certain smells can make us feel good, so, for example, we choose the bath oil with the smell that soothes our spirits. Certain essential oils can ease aching muscles and relax a tired body. We can find such oils in some 'conventional' soaps, bath oils, skin creams and lotions. When we use such things, we are, in a sense, practising aromatherapy, even if we do not call it that. When we have a cold, we can make use of eucalyptus oil – a few drops on a handkerchief can be sniffed from time to time to clear a stuffy nose. Teenagers can use tea-tree oil, or preparations containing tea-tree oil, to treat spots. It is all aromatherapy. When we sniff the flowers that we are choosing for a bouquet, enjoy the fresh scent of pine on a forest walk or pick fresh herbs from the garden for cooking – enjoying the pungent aroma that is given off by the bruised leaves of the plants – we are experiencing aromatherapy.

People have had more detailed knowledge of the secrets of the treatment now called aromatherapy for many centuries. Long before medical science was able to call upon the services of chemists, people were using extracts from plants and trees in herbal medicine, in the prevention of disease and in religious and public ceremonies all over the world.

As medical science has progressed, there has been a certain tendency for the real proven benefits of plant-based medicine to be overlooked in favour of artificial substitutes. In spite of the fact that some of the most commonly used drugs, such as digoxin, were developed from plants and are still made from plant derivatives, many people are sceptical about herbal medicine and even more dubious about the therapeutic possibilities of aromatherapy, which, after all, is also plant-based. Perhaps it is because doctors do not study aromatherapy at medical school. Perhaps it is because aromatherapy treatments do not come in the same ready-prepared and measured doses as conventional medical treatments – pills to be swallowed or fluids to be injected. There is certainly a measure of doubt in the minds of some people that something that is applied externally, as essential oils are for the most part, can have a real effect on the internal workings of the body. Nonetheless, those who take the time to find out more about aromatherapy and to try it for themselves are rarely disappointed. Aromatherapy is age-old rather than New Age, and it has many benefits to offer.

The holistic approach

Aromatherapy is a holistic form of treatment. A skilled aromatherapist will always take a patient's history in some detail. The aim is to treat the whole person rather than the symptoms alone. This approach has three benefits. Firstly, it can help patients, perhaps for the first time in years, to take a good look at themselves, their lifestyles, their states of mind, including attitudes to themselves and to their lives, and the mental and physical demands that are made on them. (Many people pay no attention to their own health until something goes wrong.) Thus made more self-aware, patients are given the chance to see beyond their symptoms, to increase their self-knowledge and to look towards ways of improving their general mental and physical wellbeing, which in turn will encourage the body to increase its ability to heal itself and combat further disease.

The second benefit of the holistic approach is that it enables the aromatherapist to look more closely at the patient, rather than just at any specific problems with which the patient has presented, to try to establish better the root causes of any ailments and thus to treat the patient rather than the symptoms alone. If the symptoms of any disease are alleviated but the cause of these symptoms is not tackled the problem is likely to return. For example, if a patient presents with a complaint that is stress-related, the aromatherapist should be able not only to help the patient to relieve the immediate symptoms but also to work with the patient to tackle the stress itself, providing both relaxing treatment and beneficial advice.

Thirdly and lastly, the holistic approach is undoubtedly

beneficial simply because it takes time. There can be little doubt of the benefits of having someone taking time to listen and to care, especially in today's world, when life seems to pass at such breakneck speed.

Aromatherapy is not a substitute for conventional medicine. No aromatherapist would claim that it is. Aromatherapists are well aware that essential oils can treat a whole catalogue of problems and also have the potential to be used in the treatment of many more, but they are not in the business of producing 'miracle' cures.

What aromatherapy does offer is a form of treatment that can do much to improve a person's general state of mental and physical wellbeing, to promote a state of balance within mind and body which will enable the individual to cope better with illness, stress and fatigue – in short, to help the body to heal itself. Aromatherapy can be used in conjunction with conventional medical treatment quite successfully, provided that both doctor and aromatherapist are aware of each other's roles in the patient's care. In many circumstances aromatherapy can offer an effective alternative to conventional forms of therapy for many physical and mental problems, an alternative that is pleasant to undergo and is free from undesirable side effects.

CAUTION

A word of warning: aromatherapy, practised responsibly at home, is safe and effective for the treatment of many minor complaints – muscular aches and pains, colds and 'flu, cuts, scrapes and spots, etc – but **the diagnosis and treatment of serious problems, or problems that you suspect might be serious, should always be left to the experts**. It is foolhardy and dangerous to 'play doctor'.

The benefits of massage

Aromatherapists use massage as their main method for the application of essential oils. Usually, a full body massage will be given, using oils that have been selected as being most appropriate for the patient. Specific areas of discomfort can also be given particular attention. Massage is an effective means of ensuring that the essential oils, which have been diluted in carrier oils, are penetrating the patient's skin. As a proportion of the volatile oils vaporises with the heat of the patient's skin, extra benefit will be gained from inhaling them.

The use of essential oils in massage, which combines application and therapeutic touch, can be beneficial in many ways.

We all, from birth onwards, appreciate the comfort that the touch of another human being can bring. When a young baby cries, its mother instinctively picks it up and soothes it in her arms, stroking and patting to bring reassurance and to help restore calm. When a child falls, the sore knee might be kissed or gently rubbed 'all better'. As we grow older, touch remains the most instinctive means of showing care and concern and offering comfort, from the sympathetic hand on another's shoulder to a warm, soothing hug. When we feel pain in our muscles, it comes naturally to us to hold, or rub, the affected part. In this way, we act as our own comforters. We are also, by giving heat and gentle friction to the area that is painful, dilating blood vessels and improving circulation to accelerate healing. (In some cases, where there is acute inflammation present, the application of heat is inappropriate, but if this is so then we are unlikely to want to touch the affected area. It will be too painful.) Massage also stimulates the lymphatic system, helping the body to rid itself of toxins.

Massage is enjoyable. It is possibly the single most pleasurable form of therapy. It relaxes the body, soothes the soul and calms the troubled mind. It is an invaluable weapon in the war against stress and can uplift the spirits of those who feel tired and depressed. Aside from the benefits that can be gained from the appropriate selection of essential oils for use in massage, the worth of the act itself can never be underestimated.

Massage can also be carried out between sexual partners, when it can be enjoyable for both the masseur and the one who is being massaged. Of course, it can be used erotically and can do much to enhance a loving sexual relationship, but massage does not have to be erotic to be pleasurable and sensual and to bring a couple closer together.

Many members of the medical professions are now appreciating the value of touch and massage. Mothers will often be advised by midwives that a gentle massage with sweet almond oil can be an effective way to soothe a fretful or 'jumpy' baby and to help cement the bond between mother and child. Babies isolated in incubators fare better when they are reassured with gentle stroking and a soothing touch. Many general practitioners are now quite willing to suggest aromatherapy and massage to patients suffering from the effects of stress. The nursing profession has also become increasingly aware of the benefits of massage and aromatherapy and its applications in their profession.

Different massage techniques can be used with different effects – details are given in the chapter on massage, *see* page 222 – but it is perfectly reasonable to state that unless the subject suffers from a condition that renders massage inadvisable, the practice of basic, gentle massage is quite safe and as long as the subject finds it enjoyable, specific health benefits apart, he or she will undoubtedly gain from it. In a world where everything moves so fast, where everybody feels the pressure to work harder and faster and longer, many people get precious few moments when they can take time, take stock and take care of themselves. The practice of massage might seem like an indulgence, but it is an indulgence that is easily justified. Unlike some of the other means by which people choose to seek pleasure and relaxation, such as alcohol, drugs and cigarettes, massage is harmless, beneficial to body and spirit, caring and bonding. We have every right to enjoy it.

Aromatherapy through time

Simple, everyday uses of many aromatic plants, such as parsley or aniseed to freshen breath, or lavender to soothe and rosemary to lift the spirits, go back many hundreds of years. The use of aromatic plants in herbal medicine is well documented and centuries old. Aromatherapy is derived from herbal medicine, using as it does a vital constituent part of the aromatic plant, i.e., the essential oil. Essential oils, like the plants from which they are extracted, also have a history of use that goes back centuries.

Many ancient civilisations appreciated the properties of the essential oils of certain plants. The Greeks, Romans, Chinese, Egyptians, Arabs, Persians and the aboriginal people of Australia, India and Africa are all known to have used essential oils as perfumes, medicines, incenses and in other ways for many hundreds of years.

Much of what we know of the ancient Egyptian people has come from the recovery of treasures and writings from the ancient tombs of the wealthy and prominent members of their society, tombs so beautifully and carefully constructed that they stand to this day. The tombs also contained the remains of the dead, meticulously preserved by the process of embalming, a process that made extensive use of essential oils such as cedarwood and myrrh. The Egyptians also used aromatic plants medicinally and for making perfumes – Cleopatra was not alone in knowing that perfumes made from certain plants had an aphrodisiac effect!

The antiseptic properties of the essential oils of certain plants were appreciated by the ancient Romans and Greeks among others. The Greeks used thyme, for example, as a fumigating agent, burning sprigs of the plant in areas where disease was present in order to prevent further spread. On the other side of the world, the Aboriginal people of Australia used eucalyptus, another strongly antiseptic plant, in much the same way. Hippocrates, the Greek physician who lived in the first century BC and whose writings and teachings showed him to be a genius of his time in the practice of medicine and surgery, made use of aromatics and of massage in his practice. Like the ancient Egyptians, the Greeks and Romans also made extensive use of aromatic plants in making perfumes and ointments, as did the Syrians and the Indian and Arab peoples.

Ayurvedic medicine, practised in India for more than three thousand years, has much in common with aromatherapy as we know it today as it uses aromatic oils in massage as one of its principal elements.

We know of the use of myrrh from various sources, but the most familiar source to most of us will be the Bible, which contains many references to precious oils and ointments. In the New Testament it is written that myrrh was brought to the infant Jesus as a birth gift by one of the three wise men from the East. Myrrh was prized in various cultures, not only as a perfume and incense ingredient but also as a disinfecting and healing agent.

Frankincense was another gift to the Christ child, another much valued ingredient of incense and medicinal oil that was used in many countries, including Arabia, China, ancient Rome and Egypt.

Basil is another particular example of a plant that has been used by many cultures for hundreds of years, for its antiseptic properties, its digestive uses and its flavour. It was used along with myrrh and incense by the ancient Egyptians for embalming. Basil oil has been used medicinally for many hundreds of years in Eastern cultures, and in ancient Rome and Greece it was used for bathing and antisepsis. In India, it has religious significance for Hindus, who believe it to be sacred to the god Krishna.

As centuries passed and people travelled farther, different cultures imparted their secrets to one another and knowledge spread. The uses of aromatic plants and the art of distillation to make them yield their precious essential oils became known far and wide across the world.

Aromatic plants and trees also spread from country to country, making it possible for people from countries where the plants were not indigenous to access their potential more easily. The crusaders in the twelfth century did much to spread the knowledge of the art of perfumery in Europe. In the Middle Ages perfumes imported from other countries became increasingly used in Great Britain. In times when personal hygiene was virtually non-existent and people rarely washed, the exotic perfumes brought from countries afar were much appreciated for their ability to mask other, less pleasant odours. The disinfectant properties of aromatic plants were also appreciated and brought into use in times of typhoid, cholera and plague.

Through the centuries, knowledge of herbal medicine increased and, in conjunction with this, knowledge of many of the uses of essential oils distilled from aromatic plants. Herbs formed the basis of the doctors' medical armoury. Essential oils were used and appreciated by two distinct professions: the medical profession and the perfumers. Each had its own band of scientists working to analyse the properties of the essential oils and ways in which to use them. The perfume and cosmetics industry grew increasingly sophisticated, and the chemists working in the field of medicine steadily worked on analysis of the chemical constituents of essential oils, identifying them and striving to replicate them in artificial preparations.

Gradually, through the eighteenth century and beyond, medical science moved on in this direction and, increasingly, doctors and chemists began to make use of chemical alternatives to traditional medicines. Whereas herbal medicine had been quite readily accessible to the average person, the new medicine was not. Doctors and scientists were now in charge. Gradually, the average man in the street came to rely more upon the professional 'medicine men' than upon the knowledge that had been passed down through families for years. Herbal medicine was now old-fashioned. Indeed, by the twentieth century, it was viewed by many with suspicion.

The specific art of aromatherapy as it is practised nowadays owes a great deal to the work of the French. The first of these were Chamberland, Meunier and Cadeac who carried out research towards the end of the nineteenth century on the efficacy of essential oils as antibacterial agents. Then in the late 1920s a French chemist called Rene Gattefosse coined the term 'aromatherapy' for the first time. He had discovered, quite by accident, that lavender oil seemed to have a beneficial effect on burnt skin. He burnt his hand while working in his laboratory and instinctively applied the nearest liquid that was to hand to ease the pain. It was lavender oil. He noticed that his hand healed remarkably quickly and that scarring was minimised. This prompted him to carry out further tests on other essential oils, and he was intrigued to find the range of medicinal properties of these oils, both in the prevention and treatment of disease. He predicted that much could be achieved if their potential was realised.

In the 1940s, another Frenchman, called Jean Valnet, a surgeon who took inspiration from Gattefosse's work, became absorbed in the subject and carried out a great deal of research of his own. He had already discovered, in the course of his work as a military surgeon during the Second World War, that essential oils were invaluable for their antiseptic properties and in the treatment of wounds. He also came to realise that essential oils worked not only on the body but also on the psychological state of the individual. He became intrigued by the possibilities that this held for the treatment of some kinds of psychiatric illness. Further work with aromatics led to the publication of a book in the 1960s, entitled

Aromatherapie. Many regard Gattefosse and Valnet as the 'fathers' of modern aromatherapy.

Another very important figure in the field, contemporary with Valnet, was Marguerite Maury, an Austrian chemist and beautician who did much to establish aromatherapy in Europe both for its cosmetic and for its medicinal applications. She was particularly interested in using essential oils in massage.

Interest in aromatherapy has been growing over time. It is true, however, that most people are still completely reliant on over-the-counter cosmetics and medical preparations that have been purchased at a pharmacy or prescribed by a doctor and consequently know little of the true potential of plants and their essences. Nevertheless, interest continues to grow to such an extent that large companies have spotted the potential in the market and now essential oils and aromatherapy products can be purchased in most high street pharmacies. Although for the most part these products are intended for cosmetic use, it is now easy for the individual to find relevant literature for information on the subject and on the essential oils for personal use. Aromatherapists worldwide have established professional organisations with their own training courses and qualifications, both for those people who wish to practise professionally and for those whose interest remains at a personal level.

We have every reason to be grateful to the medical and pharmacological sciences and the enormous advances that have been made in these fields, but it would be a pity to overlook the enormous benefits that 'alternative' – and ancient – therapies, such as aromatherapy, can bring. The upsurge of interest in aromatherapy in recent times has already gone some way to redress the balance. More and more people are beginning to see its value, both when used in conjunction with conventional medicine and sometimes as a useful and often pleasanter alternative to drug treatment.

Scientific research into the precise effects of individual oils and their chemical elements is continuing and there is much to hope for – the full potential of aromatherapy is yet to be realised.

The nature of essential oils

Essential oils are all extractions from living plants and trees, whether cultivated or wild. It is the essential oil that gives the plant its distinctive smell and, if the plant is edible, its flavour. Essential oils are extracted from different parts of different plants. Some plants, such as jasmine, yield their oils from the flower; others, such as rosemary, do so from the leaves. Other kinds of plant contain essential oils in their seeds, in their roots or, in the case of some trees, in the wood or bark. Essential oils can also be extracted from some aromatic grasses. There are currently more than two hundred plants and trees from which essential oils are extracted, although not all these essential oils can be used therapeutically.

In some plants, the essential oil is contained in microscopic quantities whilst in others there are more generous amounts. Similarly, some essential oils are much easier to extract than others. Jasmine, a flower much prized by the perfume industry for its heady scent, yields, with reluctance, notoriously small quantities of its precious essential oil. For every ounce of oil that is produced, one thousand times that weight of flowers must be used. On the other hand, three different essential oils can be extracted from citrus fruit trees: the flowers, the leaves and the skin of the fruit all contain essential oils. It is particularly easy to extract the oil from the skin and pith of the fruit. They are squeezed by hand or (much more frequently nowadays) in a mechanical press to express the vital juices.

The herbs that are particularly enjoyable to touch in the garden, giving off a waft of aroma when their leaves are rubbed between the fingers, release minute quantities of their essential oils into the atmosphere and onto the skin. Some of these oils have particularly lingering perfumes. Lavender oil is like this. Old-fashioned lavender bags, filled with dried lavender flower heads, make long-lasting and effective drawer fresheners.

Essential oils are volatile substances that evaporate easily when heated. They all contain a complex combination of many different chemicals which give them their individual qualities and effects. Terpenes are an important component in the citrus oils, for example. It is the terpene content in these oils that makes them prone to more rapid oxidisation and deterioration than some other essential oils. Most essential oils are high in alcohols, which give them their antiseptic properties. Esters, another group of chemicals found in many essential oils, have a sedative effect. Essential oils that contain high proportions of phenols will have antibacterial qualities. The chemical make-up of each herb is also dependent to some extent on the place where it has been cultivated. Thus two samples of the same herb, grown in different places and under different conditions, can produce oils that have a slightly different chemical make-up.

Not all essential oils are suitable for therapeutic use. Some are highly toxic. It is interesting to note that the essential oils of certain herbs and spices that are widely used for culinary purposes fall into this category. For example, mustard is considered an essential condiment in kitchens all over the world. The essential oil extracted from mustard seeds, however, is extremely toxic. It has no therapeutic use whatsoever. The leaves of the herb chervil make a refreshing addition to salads, and the juice obtained fresh from the leaves is used in herbal medicine for its healing properties, but essential oil of chervil is toxic, an irritant and a possible carcinogen.

Some essential oils are free-flowing liquids, whilst others are more viscous and some are solid or semi-solid until heated. Essential oils dissolve easily in alcohol and oil but not in water. The volatility of essential oils, their swift evaporation when exposed to heat, is a property that is exploited both in the extraction processes and in the therapeutic use of the oils.

Essential oils are very concentrated and the vast majority of them irritate the skin when used neat. Some are quite toxic unless well diluted. Used in appropriate dilution, however, they all have their own distinct thera-peutic qualities, and many of them can be used and en-joyed quite safely and with beneficial effects in a do-mestic environment by 'lay' people.

CAUTION

- As a general rule, essential oils should never be ap-plied neat to the skin. Exceptions to this rule are tea tree and lavender.
- Essential oils are flammable – extremely so. If you use them in a burner, put a few drops in water – not oil – in the bowl of the burner and allow the perfume to enter the atmosphere through evaporation.
- Although some practitioners will occasionally prescribe essential oils by mouth, this is the exception rather then the rule. **When using essential oils at home, use them for external application only.** Unless they have been specifically prescribed by a qualified person, it should be assumed that they are not safe to be in-gested. Some essential oils are very toxic indeed if swallowed. Some oils have benefits in the treatment of certain oral ailments, when used as a mouthwash or gargle in recommended dilution, but even so should **never** be swallowed.

- If you are storing essential oils at home, make sure that they are kept well out of the reach of children.
- Always seek the advice of a trained aromatherapist if you wish to use essential oils during pregnancy or on babies and young children.
- If using homeopathy or herbal medidcine seek the advice of the relevant practitioner as well as that of an aromatherapist
- Some medical conditions conta-indicate the use of certain essential oils and/or massage. If you suffer from any kind of medical condition always check with your doctor first and always consult a trained aromatherapist before you use essential oils.

The Extraction of Essential Oils

Steam distillation

Essential oils are extracted from different parts of different plants. The most common method of oil extraction is by steam distillation. In countries where the source plants are grown, stills are more often than not kept very close to the cultivation areas to ensure the optimum freshness of the plants used for distillation. The appropriate part of the plant – seeds, leaves, stems, flowers or a combination of more than one of these – is compacted into the first container in the still. Steam is then passed through the still and the essential oil evaporates with the heat of the steam. The evaporated essential oil rises and passes, with the steam, through a condenser and into a collecting vessel where cooling takes place. When the essential oil and water are cooled, the oil will separate from the water and can be siphoned off the top.

Some plants, such as jasmine, do not respond well to steam distillation as the heat is too intense to preserve the odour. Two different methods of extraction are used in cases such as this. What is produced by these processes is not, strictly speaking, an essential oil but an absolute.

Enfleurage

The first process, enfleurage, is still practised by some perfumeries in France, sometimes only for demonstration purposes for the benefit of visiting tourists, but it is more or less obsolete elsewhere. It is labour-intensive and extremely slow, but it produces a very high quality jasmine absolute that is strong and pure. The jasmine flowers are spread out by hand on glass trays containing special fat. The trays are then stacked up and left lying to give the oil time to penetrate the fat. The process is then repeated, the used flowers being lifted off and replaced with fresh ones, until the fat is absolutely saturated with essential oil. The saturated fat is known as a pomade. When the pomade is ready it is then processed with alcohol to separate the jasmine absolute. The residue fat in the enfleurage process need not be wasted. It retains some of the odour of the jasmine and can be used for soap manufacture.

Solvent extraction

The second method of extracting jasmine absolute is by

solvent extraction; some other plants are also processed in a similar way.

The flowers (or relevant parts of the plant) are macerated and mixed in a container with a solvent such as hexane. The extract is then heated to vaporise the solvent that now contains the essential oil and plant waxes. When the solvent has evaporated, what remains is known as a concrete, roughly half absolute and half plant wax.

After cooling, further processing of the concrete with alcohol separates the absolute from the wax.

Resinoids are also produced by solvent extraction from gums and resinous materials. Some resinoids can be further processed with alcohol to produce an absolute.

Carbon dioxide extraction

Carbon dioxide extraction is a relatively new process compared to the others but may become a method preferred to solvent extraction over time. There is some concern about the amounts of solvent that remain in the concretes and absolutes after solvent extraction and the use of carbon dioxide avoids this problem.

Essential Oils at Work

Essential oils work on two distinct levels, the psycho-logical and the physical.

Imagine some of your favourite aromas. How do they make you feel? Certain smells can trigger happy memo-ries of places or people, taking you back to early child-hood, to the kitchen at home, perhaps, or to a particular person, such as your mother. Some smells will make you think of a certain time of year – the freshness of spring or the sun-baked days of summer. Other smells that you find enjoyable might be harder to explain – they simply make you feel good. If you are trying to sell your house, the estate agent may well tell you to put a pot of coffee on the stove before prospective buyers come to view, or make some bread or cakes to fill the house with the scent of fresh baking. Smell is a primitive and pow-erful sense. Not only can it alert us to danger (think of the odour of meat that has gone bad or the smell of a gas leak), it can also trigger memories, alter our moods and either attract us to, or put us off, potential mates. Recent research has shown that human beings have not yet become so sophisticated that the sense of smell has become irrelevant in the process of sexual attraction. No matter how beautiful, intelligent and witty you might be, the object of your heart's desire will still be affected by your own, very individual smell.

The fragrant essential oils of many plants can have quite a powerful effect on the mind, altering mood quite noticeably when they are inhaled. This is what makes aromatherapy particularly useful in the treatment of mood disturbances such as depression and anxiety and the consequent effects these problems have on the individual's ability to function properly. Some oils will have a definite sedative, calming effect, whilst others are useful for their stimulant properties, increasing mental and physical energy. Certain oils are particularly good at helping to focus the mind; such oils are often burned in incense, as an aid to meditation. Some oils will stimulate sexual appetites and can be used as aphrodisiacs.

It is still something of a mystery as to how the smells of essential oils can affect emotion and mood so profoundly. The odours of the oils are taken up by receptor cells within the nasal cavity which are connected, via the olfactory nerve, to the limbic system in the brain – the part of the brain that controls emotion and memory. Whether the response of the brain is entirely because of the particular chemical make-up of the oils is uncertain, but the brain is stimulated by the smells to release certain neurochemicals into the bloodstream. Some neurochemicals, such as serotonin, promote relaxation and can induce sleep while others have a stimulating effect. Endorphins are another group of chemicals that can be produced in response to essential oil odours. These are opiate-like substances that inhibit pain and induce a feeling of wellbeing. They are, in short, 'feel-good' chemicals.

On a purely physiological level, different essential oils, according to their individual chemical make-up, will each have their own specific effects on the internal workings of the body.

There are three ways by which essential oils can enter the body. The first of these is by inhalation, which allows for the oil molecules to enter the body through the tiny capillaries supplying the respiratory organs.

Essential oils can also be absorbed into the body by skin absorption – by bathing in hot water to which oils have been added, by applying essential oils in topical preparations or in compresses, and by massage.

The third means by which essential oils can enter

the body is by ingestion. Some qualified aromatherapists will prescribe the use of some essential oils in this way, but on the whole massage is the preferred method of treatment. **Ingestion of essential oils is potentially very dangerous and should never be tried in the home.**

One property that many essential oils have in common is the ability to stimulate the body's immune system, that is, to encourage the body to heal itself. Antiseptic and bactericidal properties are also common to most essential oils eucalyptus oil and tea-tree oil being particularly useful in this respect. Many oils (tea-tree oil falls into this category too) have antiviral and/or fungicidal properties.

Antibiotics have for many years been an invaluable weapon in the war against many diseases, but overuse has led to an increase in antibiotic-resistant strains of bacteria. Antibiotics also kill off many other, harmless and/or beneficial bacteria, leading to problems such as *Candida albicans*, or thrush, and they can have unpleasant side effects. When suffering from a relatively minor infection that is likely to respond well to treatment with essential oils, it makes a lot of sense to choose this option rather than resorting to antibiotics.

Massage

This is the main method of treatment used by qualified aromatherapists. Massage allows for a combination of the beneficial effects of the absorption of essential oils through the skin and those of therapeutic massage; as the therapist's hands work on the patient's body, circulation and lymphatic drainage will be stimulated and the patient's muscles will relax. At the same time, helped by the heat caused by the friction of the therapist's hands on the patient's body, the oil molecules can enter the body through the skin and will start to take effect on the patient. The patient will gain further benefit as he or she breathes in the fragrance. While not all the oils that are used by aromatherapists in practice are recommended for use in the home, there is nonetheless a wide variety of essential oils that can be used perfectly safely by people who lack the aromatherapists' expertise but want to derive some benefit and pleasure from home massage. Massage techniques are detailed in the relevant chapter (*see* page 222). Essential oils for massage can be diluted in a base oil, either singly or blended with one or two other harmonising, synergistic, oils. Base oils suitable for aromatherapy include almond oil, avocado oil, jojoba oil, and wheatgerm oil – *see* Selecting and

Using Base Oils, page 66. Doubtless you will have your own preferences, but each has its own qualities; avocado, for example, is beneficial to dry skin. Try to establish that the base oil you intend to use has been cold-pressed and preferably is organic and thus as pure and chemical-free as possible. When it comes to the dilution quantities, 1–3 per cent essential oil to base oil is generally a safe option, but if you have any doubts, you can check with an aromatherapist.

Inhalation

Steam inhalation is used mostly for the treatment of respiratory disorders. To prepare, fill a fairly large bowl with very hot water and add a few drops of the essential oil, or oils, of choice. Drape a towel over your head and 'tent' it all round the bowl then breathe in the scented steam deeply. Continue treatment for a few minutes, but stop if you feel too hot. Place the bowl on a surface at a height that does not require you to bend over it. Raising your head suddenly, especially if you have been bending over, might cause dizziness. Steam inhalation is beneficial to respiratory ailments in two ways. Firstly, the steam moistens the airways and helps to loosen mucus and clear blocked sinuses. Secondly, the essential oil vapours will enter the bloodstream rapidly and work their own individual 'magic', whether this is to promote expectoration or fight off infection.

Dry inhalation is also beneficial with certain aromatic oils and can be useful in the treatment of asthmatics, whose lungs may be irritated by steam inhalation. A few drops of essential oil can be applied to a handkerchief that is then held a few inches under the patient's nose as he or she breathes in. Alternatively, a few drops can be placed on the pillow (away from the eyes) at bedtime. Eucalyptus oil is a favourite for use in dry inhalation to ease the discomfort of blocked noses. Lavender oil on the pillow will help promote restful sleep.

If you are treating oily skin with aromatic steam, it is pleasant to finish treatment with a refreshing splash of rose water, which will tone the skin. Steam treatment is not recommended if you suffer from thread veins or if you have any inflammatory skin condition.

Steam facial

A steam facial, taken in much the same way as a steam inhalation, can be a very effective way of opening the pores and cleansing the skin, particularly skin that is prone to oiliness and spots. There are several essential oils that can be used in this way. It is pleasant and refreshing to finish off the treatment with a splash of rose water.

CAUTION
Do not use steam facials if you have broken veins or very sensitive skin.

Bathing
Aromatic bathing is a wonderful way to treat yourself and do yourself some good at the same time. Bathing with essential oils allows for the oil to be absorbed firstly through the skin and secondly, as the oils evaporate in the steam from the bath, through inhalation of the fragrant steamy atmosphere in the bathroom. This form of treatment has the advantage that, unlike massage, it can be done without the help of another person.

Run a hot bath with the door and windows closed and add a few drops (3–10, depending on the oil or oils of choice) of essential oil into the water. Make sure that the oil is thoroughly dispersed in the water to avoid the possibility of concentrated amounts of oil coming into contact with the skin. Prolonged and frequent use of essential oils can damage the surface of some baths; make sure the bath is thoroughly cleaned out afterwards. To avoid problems with sensitive skin, and also to preserve your bath, dilute the essential oil in a base oil before you add it to the bath. You can also dilute the essential oil in milk.

Choose your essential oil or oils according to the desired effect you wish to achieve – rosemary to revive your flagging spirits, perhaps, or chamomile to set you up for a good night's sleep. Take all the time you need – lie back in the water and breathe deeply – an aromatic bath should be a very pleasurable experience.

NOTE
Don't use soaps, bath oils or shampoos in an aromatic bath. If you want to clean yourself with soap, or wash your hair, do this beforehand – have a quick shower or wash before you run your aromatic bath.

An aromatic footbath is also a soothing and refreshing way of treating tired, aching feet and will benefit not only your feet but also your whole body. If you only have a shower at home, treat yourself to a footbath from time to time. Lavender, peppermint and rosemary are particularly beneficial at the end of a long day. Footbaths can also help to warm cold feet, and the addition of appropriate oils will stimulate the circulation.

Full immersion bathing is not advisable with some oils

that can irritate the skin and/or mucous membranes. *See* A–Z of Plants and their Essential Oils, page 72.

Sitz baths

Sitz baths, or hip baths, are particularly beneficial in the treatment of menstrual disorders, thrush, cystitis, haemorrhoids and constipation. When treating haemorrhoids or vaginal thrush keep the water around body temperature, but otherwise the water should be quite hot. Tea-tree oil is particularly useful in the treatment of thrush.

NOTE

As with full immersion bathing, sitz bathing is not appropriate with some essential oils. *See* A–Z of Plants and their Essential Oils, page 72.

Compresses

Some problems respond well to treatment with compresses, made by soaking cloths or towels in either hot or ice-cold water – whichever is appropriate – and adding a few drops of essential oil. Cold compresses are useful for treating headaches, fever and pain from recent bruising or muscle strain. Hot compresses, applied to the relevant parts of the body, can alleviate menstrual cramping and muscle and joint pain and can be particularly soothing for chronic pain caused by arthritis and rheumatism. Hot compresses can also be used to treat boils.

To prepare a compress, fill a bowl with either hot or iced water, according to your needs. Soak a folded cloth in the water and wring it out. Add three or four drops of essential oil to the water in the bowl and swirl it round to disperse it thoroughly. Lay your cloth lightly back on the surface of the water, then wring out again and apply to the affected part for treatment.

If you are using a hot compress, place some polythene or clingfilm over the compress with another cloth on top. This will help to retain the heat.

If you are treating headache with a cold compress, make sure that the compress is well wrung out and will not drip. It is important that the essential oil is kept away from the eyes.

Mouthwashes

Some essential oils can be added to warm water and used as mouthwashes or gargles to combat gum inflammation, bad breath, oral thrush and mouth ulcers. *See* A–Z of Plants and their Essential Oils, page 72. In order to avoid irritation of the mouth, the oil should be first diluted in a small amount of alcohol – vodka is generally recommended. Add two drops of essential oil to a teaspoon of vodka and mix into half a glass of warm water to prepare your mouthwash. Tea-tree oil is safe to add to warm water without alcohol, but this is the exception.

CAUTION
Mouthwashes should never be swallowed.

Skin care
There is a variety of ways in which appropriate essential oils can be used to benefit the skin. Facial massage with essential oils diluted in a base oil will stimulate the circulation, help to improve skin tone and impart the individual benefits of the essential oils to the skin. Dry, flaky and ageing skin will derive particular benefit from this treatment. Careful choice of an appropriate carrier oil will make the treatment even more effective (*see* Selecting Base Oils, page 66).

Steam facials (*see* page 37) are an effective way of cleansing and treating skins prone to oiliness or acne.

Essential oils can also be added to unscented creams or lotions for application to the skin or, for the treatment of fungal infections and cold sores, diluted in a little alcohol (isopropyl alcohol is available from most chemists) before application to the affected area.

Neat application is inadvisable for most essential oils; but tea-tree oil and lavender oil are safe to use in this way. Tea-tree oil can be applied to spots. Lavender oil can be used on a variety of skin traumas: minor cuts, burns and scalds and insects bites and stings.

Lemon oil can be used to treat verrucas and warts but the surrounding skin should be protected with petroleum jelly.

Hair care

There are quite a few essential oils that can be used on the hair for a variety of reasons. Tea-tree oil, for example, will help in the treatment of dandruff. Rosemary will help to stimulate hair growth and condition the hair. Dilute in a carrier oil as for massage and rub well into the scalp. The oil can be left on the scalp for an hour or so. Wrap a towel around the head and leave, then wash as normal.

Vaporisers, diffusers, room sprays, burners

All the above may be used to add fragrance to a room

with essential oils, letting the occupants benefit from smelling the odours that are given off. Certain oils can also be used as fumigating or disinfecting agents in this way, preventing the spread of disease. Others will make effective insect-repellents (*see* A–Z of Plants and Essential Oils).

There is quite a selection of devices for fragrancing a room with essential oils, including electrically powered devices. Burners (a saucer-shaped dish above a candle in a holder) should always be used with extreme care. Use only the type of candle that is advised in the instructions or the whole dish might become overheated. Never place the oils neat in the burner dish: always float them in water.

Electric vaporisers can be bought in many large pharmacies. Make sure that they are suitable for use with essential oils.

Ring burners are also available: ring-shaped dishes that are fixed above a light bulb. Never allow any essential oil to drip onto the light bulb when it is hot.

One of the easiest and safest ways to scent a room with essential oils is to fill a bowl with boiling water, add some essential oils, and place it in the room with doors and windows closed for a while. Alternatively, place a bowl of water with essential oils added on top of a central heating radiator.

You can make your own room spray quite easily with a plant spray, some water and a few drops of the oils of your choice.

CAUTION

With one or two exceptions, the application of undiluted essential oil onto the skin is strictly inadvisable. Exceptions are lavender oil, which can be used as an antiseptic on cuts and scrapes, and tea-tree oil, which is useful in the treatment of spots and can be dabbed onto blemishes neat. Oil of lemon can be used on warts and verrucas but the surrounding skin should be well protected with petroleum jelly. If you notice any skin irritation after using any essential oils, discontinue treatment immediately. It is possible to become sensitised to some essential oils that you might have been using without any problems beforehand.

If you have sensitive skin, it is advisable to carry out a patch test with any essential oil that you would like to use. Dilute the oil in a base oil as you would for a massage blend and apply to a small area on the inside of your wrist. If you notice any redness or irritation within the next few hours, you should not use the oil.

Blending Essential Oils

If you make an appointment with a trained aroma-therapist, you will find that he or she will take time to ask you in some detail about your lifestyle and your medical history. Diet and exercise, sleep patterns, stress levels, mood, bowel habits, menstrual cycle if you are a woman – all have some relevance as they will help the therapist to draw up as complete a picture as possible of you, the patient, rather than 'it', the problem for which you are seeking help. All the information will help in the selection of oils that are likely to be the most beneficial to you as an individual and as a whole.

You will notice, as you read the A–Z of Plants and their Essential Oils, that several oils may share the same basic property; for example, quite a few have a relaxing effect, while others act as antidepressants. Within each group, there will be one or more that are particularly appropriate for individual cases, when other relevant factors are taken into consideration. Depression, for example, can manifest itself in different ways. A person who feels anxious, agitated and has trouble sleeping at night should be treated differently from one whose depression manifests itself in flatness of mood and lethargy.

When the aromatherapist selects which oils to use, he or she will also be considering which ones work in harmony with each other, both for fragrance and for effect. A successful, harmonious blend of oils that work well in combination with one another is known as a synergistic blend. As many as seven oils may be used in combination, but the art of blending is one that takes quite a lot of practice. When preparing blends at home, it is generally better to keep it simple at first and work with no more than four essential oils at a time. If you work with simple blends initially, you will gradually build up a repertoire of blends that you enjoy using. Write everything down as you go along – mistakes should be remembered so that you do not repeat them – and then, gradually, you will find that you are able to add to and alter your recipes. Successful blending takes a combination of time, patience, expertise and intuition. Remember, however, that it is not necessarily the case that complicated blends are more effective. Often, keeping it simple is better.

Mix your blends in small quantities. Once essential oils are mixed in base oils, they do not last as long. It is better to work with small quantities, making fresh blends each time, than to make up large amounts if you are not certain whether you are going to use a particular blend again in the immediate future. Blending small amounts also makes mistakes less costly.

In order to achieve a blend that is approximately a 2 per cent dilution, use six drops of essential oil to every tablespoon of base oil. For even smaller quantities, use two drops of essential oil to one teaspoon of base. Remember that some base oils have their own distinctive qualities; if you make a blend of essential oils in almond oil, for example, a light base oil that is virtually odourless and suitable for general use, it will not be the same if you use a different base the next time.

Blending guide

With time and practice, you will be able to build up your own 'menu' of favourite blends. The following may help you in your initial selection of essential oils in blends that you prepare. As a general rule, like blends well with like, so the spice oils can be blended with each other, the oils from the same plant family – for example *Labiateae* which includes basil, clary sage and hyssop – will work quite well together, the woody oils can be used in combination with each other, and so on. There are other broad guidelines that can be followed as well: citrus oils, for example, have an odour that is short-lived, but they blend well with the woody oils, whose fragrance is more lingering, so you can make blends that have a fragrance that changes in quality as time goes on. Perfumers consider that a good perfume should have a top note, a middle note and a base note. The top note is the shortest-lived, but probably makes the first impression. The base note is the longest-lived, the last lingering element of the fragrant blend. The middle note is the basis around which the fragrance is built – the substance of the perfume. Thus, in an aromatherapy blend, each oil will have its own distinctive qualities but, put together with others, will form part of a dynamic fragrance, changing its impressions on the individual all the time. Whilst this might sound a little complicated to the novice, it does serve to make the point that it is more than the instant first impression that counts when blending oils. If you are trying out a blend for the first time give it time. What is your first feeling about the blend? What comes through immediately after the first impression? What is it like after half an hour or an hour? How does it change?

Remember also that the therapeutic qualities of the oils that you choose should complement each other. Think of the outcome you are hoping to achieve.

Finally, if you are intending to give a massage to another person or are mixing a bath blend for the benefit of another individual, his or her likes and dislikes cannot be ignored. No matter how you might feel about the blend that you are making, it is the recipient who counts. In order for that person to get the maximum benefit from the oils, the blend should smell good to him or her.

Many books have been written on the subject of aromatherapy that give specific recipes for the treatment of certain problems, and these are very useful indeed, especially if you are looking for a 'springboard' to start you off practising aromatherapy at home. They will also give valuable advice on which oils, used therapeutically, are best to use in combination with one another.

The following is not a therapeutic guide. It is meant simply as a guide to some of the oils that are likely to work most successfully with one another in a blend. The proportions will vary according to individual taste.

Angelica
Blends well with citrus oils, clary sage, patchouli, vetiver.

Basil
Blends well with bergamot, citronella, chamomile, clary sage, geranium, lavender, lemongrass, lime, marjoram, peppermint, rose.

Bay
Blends well with citrus oils, clary sage, cypress, hyssop, lavender, myrtle, rosemary.

Benzoin
Blends well with black pepper, coriander, cardamom, cumin, cypress, frankincense, jasmine, juniper, myrrh, peppermint, petitgrain.

Bergamot
Blends well with basil, cardamom, chamomile, coriander, cypress, geranium, jasmine, juniper, lavender, melissa, mimosa, myrtle, neroli, pctitgrain, sandalwood, ylang ylang.

Black pepper
Blends well with cedarwood, frankincense, juniper, lemon, marjoram, palmarosa, rosemary, sandalwood.

Cajeput
Blends well with cedarwood, eucalyptus, lavender, pine.

Cardamom
Blends well with bergamot, cedarwood, cumin, frankincense, neroli, orange, rose, sandalwood, ylang ylang.

Carrot seed
Blends well with cedarwood, citrus oils (particularly orange), geranium, mimosa.

Cedarwood
Blends well with benzoin, bergamot, black pepper, cajeput, cypress, frankincense, ginger, jasmine, juniper, lavender, myrrh, neroli, patchouli, pine, rose, rosemary, sandalwood, vetiver, ylang ylang.

Chamomile
Blends well with basil, bergamot, clary sage, jasmine, lavender, marjoram, rose, star anise.

Cinnamon leaf
Blends well with benzoin, eucalyptus, frankincense, lemon, mandarin, orange.

Citronella
Blends well with bergamot, cedarwood, geranium, lemon, mimosa, orange, pine.

Clary sage
Blends well with angelica, basil, bay, cardamom, cedarwood, coriander, frankincense, geranium, jasmine, lavender, lemon, myrtle, petigrain, rose, sandalwood, ylang ylang.

Coriander
Blends well with bergamot, carrot, citronella, clary sage, cypress, frankincense, ginger, jasmine, pine, sandalwood.

Cumin
Blends well with cardamom, coriander, lavender, rosemary, rosewood.

Cypress
Blends well with bay, benzoin, bergamot, cardamom, cedarwood, clary sage, frankincense, juniper, lavender, lemon, mandarin, marjoram, orange, sandalwood.

Dill
Blends with lemon, mandarin, neroli, orange, peppermint.

Eucalyptus
Blends well with cajeput, cedarwood, cypress, lavender, lemon, lemongrass, marjoram, peppermint, pine, rosemary, star anise, tea tree, thyme.

Fennel
Blends reasonably well with geranium, lavender, marjoram, rose, sandalwood, but many people prefer fennel used on its own because of its distinctive odour.

Frankincense
Blends well with basil, black pepper, cedarwood, cinnamon, citrus oils, geranium, ginger, myrrh, neroli, pine, sandalwood, vetiver.

Geranium
Blends well with basil, bergamot, hyssop, jasmine, juniper, lemon, lime, mandarin, marjoram, neroli, orange, patchouli, petitgrain, rose, sandalwood, tea tree.

Ginger

Blends well with cedarwood, coriander, frankincense, grapefruit, juniper, lemon, mandarin, myrtle, orange, palmarosa, patchouli, rose, rosewood, vetiver.

Grapefruit

Blends well with bergamot and other citrus oils, cardamom, cypress, geranium, ginger, lavender, neroli, palmarosa, rosemary.

Hyssop

Blends well with bay, clary sage, geranium, lavender, orange, rosemary.

Jasmine

Blends well with bergamot and other citrus oils, chamomile, clary sage, coriander, geranium, lavender, mimosa, myrtle, patchouli, peppermint, petitgrain, rose, sandalwood, vetiver, ylang ylang.

Juniper

Blends well with cedarwood, citrus oils, cypress, geranium, ginger, lavender, pine, rosemary, sandalwood, vetiver.

Lavender
Blends well with basil, bergamot, cardamom, clary sage, cumin, cedarwood, cypress, eucalyptus, geranium, grapefruit, hyssop, lemon, lemongrass, lime, marjoram, myrtle, neroli, orange, peppermint, petitgrain, rosemary, tea tree.

Lemon
Blends well with angelica, bay, benzoin, black pepper, citronella, citrus oils, eucalyptus, fennel, geranium, ginger, jasmine, juniper, lavender, neroli, peppermint, ylang ylang.

Lemongrass
Blends well with basil, coriander, eucalyptus, lavender, peppermint, rosemary, thyme, vetiver.

Lime
Blends well with basil, citronella, citrus oils, clary sage, lavender, neroli, nutmeg, rosemary.

Mandarin
Blends well with bergamot and other citrus oils, coriander, cinnamon, cumin, clary sage, geranium, juniper, lavender, nutmeg.

Marjoram

Blends well with basil, bergamot, cedarwood, chamomile, cypress, eucalyptus, geranium, lavender, melissa, orange, peppermint, rosemary, tea tree, thyme.

Melissa

Blends well with chamomile, citrus oils, geranium, jasmine, lavender, marjoram, rose, rosemary, thyme.

Mimosa

Blends well with citronella, citrus oils, coriander, jasmine, lavender, rose, sandalwood, ylang ylang.

Myrrh

Blends well with benzoin, cedarwood, cypress, frankincense, geranium, juniper, lavender, lemon, patchouli, peppermint, pine, sandalwood.

Myrtle

Blends well with bay, bergamot, clary sage, cardamom, ginger, hyssop, lavender, lime, rosemary.

Neroli
Blends well with all citrus oils, clary sage, jasmine, lavender, rosemary, rosewood.

Niaouli
Blends well with eucalyptus, lavender, rosemary, tea tree.

Nutmeg
Blends well with bay, cinnamon, clary sage, coriander, cumin, geranium, ginger, lime, mandarin, petitgrain.

Orange (sweet or bitter)
Blends well with black pepper, all citrus oils, cinnamon, clary sage, coriander, cumin, ginger, hyssop, jasmine, lavender, myrrh, neroli, nutmeg, petitgrain.

Palmarosa
Blends well with black pepper, cedarwood, geranium, jasmine, neroli, petitgrain, rose, rosewood, sandalwood.

Patchouli
Blends well with angelica, cedarwood, clary sage, geranium, neroli, nutmeg, orange, rose, rosewood, sandalwood, ylang ylang.

Peppermint
Blends well with basil, benzoin, eucalyptus, jasmine, lavender, lemon, lemongrass, marjoram, pine, rosemary.

Petitgrain
Blends well with benzoin, bergamot, clary sage, geranium, jasmine, lavender, orange, palmarosa, rosemary.

Pine
Blends well with cajeput, cedarwood, eucalyptus, juniper, lavender, lemon, marjoram, niaouli, peppermint, rosemary, tea tree.

Rose
Blends well with basil, benzoin, bergamot, chamomile, clary sage, geranium, jasmine, lavender, patchouli, sandalwood, star anise, ylang ylang.

Rosemary
Blends well with basil, black pepper, hyssop, lavender, lemongrass, orange, peppermint, petitgrain, pine, tea tree.

Rosewood
Blends well with all citrus oils, jasmine, lavender, neroli, patchouli, rose, sandalwood, ylang ylang.

Sandalwood
Blends well with bergamot, cedarwood, geranium, jasmine, lavender, mimosa, palmarosa, patchouli, rosewood, vetiver, ylang ylang.

Star anise
Blends well with chamomile, cinnamon, eucalyptus, lavender, orange, pine, rose, rosemary.

Tarragon
Blends well with basil, pine.

Tea tree
Blends well with black pepper, clary sage, coriander, cumin, eucalyptus, geranium, lavender, lemon, marjoram, nutmeg, pine, rosemary, thyme.

Thyme
Blends well with bergamot, eucalyptus, lavender, lemon, marjoram, melissa, pine, rosemary, tea tree.

Vetiver

Blends well with angelica, clary sage, jasmine, lavender, patchouli, rose, sandalwood, ylang ylang.

Ylang ylang

Blends well with bergamot, cedarwood, clary sage, jasmine, lemon, mimosa, patchouli, rose, sandalwood, vetiver.

Storage of Essential Oils and Blended Oils

Essential oils are best bought in small quantities. It may seem more economical to buy in larger quantities, but the more often a bottle is opened and the oil is exposed to the air, the more it will deteriorate. A larger bottle of oil may thus go 'off' before it is finished. Essential oils, kept properly, will last for quite some time; most will be usable for up to two years although a few, such as citrus oils, have a shorter life.

Store your blends in small coloured glass bottles, carefully labelled. The 'shelf life' of blends is shorter than that of essential oils. It will vary according to the oils that you have used, but two to three months is generally the norm.

Keep essential oils and blended oils in a cool, dark place; the refrigerator is ideal, but if you have very young children who have access to the fridge, a safer alternative is a locked cupboard in an unheated room. Alternatively, you can use a childproof lock on the fridge door. Some oils will become more viscous in colder conditions; remove these from the fridge when required and allow them to come back to room temperature and they will be ready for use as normal.

NOTE

If you do intend storing your essential oils in the fridge, it is advisable to keep them in a tightly sealed container. Once the oils have been opened, it is inevitable that small quantities will have dribbled onto the neck of the bottle and no matter how small the amount, the potent fragrance can spread to other foods in the fridge. Cheese with a hint of lavender is not to everyone's taste!

Purchase of essential oils

There are several places where you can buy a wide variety of essential oils. Many pharmacies now stock them, as well as herbalists and centres of complementary medicine. You can also order essential oils by post from some suppliers. Choose a source that provides information, or is willing to provide information, about the oils that it supplies – the keeping qualities of the oils, their uses, dilution advice, safety precautions, etc. A knowledgeable source is more likely to be a reliable source.

It is also advisable that you purchase oils that have a tamper-proof seal on the bottles. The more often an essential oil is exposed to the air, the more quickly it oxidises. For this reason, you do not want to buy oils that might have been opened several times by curious customers taking a sniff!

As with food products, there is a growing demand for essential oils to be organically produced. Reliable stockists will have a range of organically produced oils in the selection they have to offer. Check that the oils that are claimed to be organic have a logo on the bottle from an organisation such as the Soil Association (United Kingdom), which guarantees the reliability of source.

You can buy many products 'ready-made': bath oils, skin care products, etc. that claim to be aromatherapy treatments. Some (not all) of these products will *not* live up to their claims – check the ingredients carefully! Some 'aromatherapy' products will contain artificial, chemical substitutes for essential oils. These might smell similar, but they will not smell the same. Nor will they have the same effects. In addition to this, the base oil that has been used in the formulation of these products may be a mineral oil rather than a vegetable oil. Mineral oils are not suitable for aromatherapy as they are too heavy to penetrate the skin.

Finally, make sure that the essential oils you purchase are just that, essential, rather than a mixture of essential oil and base.

Selecting and Using Base Oils

There is quite a large variety of oils that you can use as base, or carrier, oils in aromatherapy. The oil you select will depend very much on personal preference and the purpose for which it is intended. The list below gives a summary of some of the many carrier oils that can be used. Individuals will always find their own favourites, whether for massage, as bath blends or for skin care.

Remember that base oils do not have an unlimited shelf life. Store in a cool dark place and do not keep for more than one year.

Almond oil

Almond oil has many advantages as a base oil and is probably a good one to keep as a stock item in your store. It is relatively inexpensive, bland and quite safe to use on most people. It is also, if cold-pressed, high in nutrients. Be cautious, however, about using almond oil on anyone with a known nut allergy, as a few unlucky sufferers will suffer a reaction to any nut oil on their skin. **Warning:** Always make sure that the subject is not allergic to nuts.

Apricot-kernel oil

Apricot kernel oil is particularly light, which makes it suitable for use on the skin of the face. It has no detectable smell. It is, however, quite expensive.

Avocado oil

Avocado oil is very rich in nutrients, in particular vitamin E, which makes it a good preservative, helping to keep essential oils that are blended with it fresh. Avocado oil is green in colour, and because of its heaviness people often choose to mix it with another base oil in a proportion of one to ten. It is good for the treatment of dry skin but is not suitable for those whose skin has a tendency to be oily.

Coconut oil

Coconut oil is particularly well suited to hair and scalp treatment. It imparts a lovely sheen to the hair. It is also very soothing and nourishing on dry skin.

Grapeseed oil

Grapeseed oil is light and virtually odourless. It can be used on its own as a base oil, or alternatively can be used as the main base to which a smaller amount (generally 10 per cent) of another richer base oil has been added.

Jojoba oil

Like coconut oil, jojoba oil is solid and waxy at room temperature, but it has the benefit of good skin penetration and is also anti-inflammatory, making it soothing on hot, irritated skin. It can be mixed with other base oils once heated, in one to ten proportions, and many people will go for this option because of the expense of undiluted jojoba.

Olive oil

Olive oil is suitable for use in the treatment of scalp conditions and dry skin. It does, however, have quite a distinctive colour and odour of its own, which not everyone will appreciate, and it is quite heavy. Some people will find it preferable to use olive oil in combination with another, lighter base oil.

Disregard the cheaper varieties of olive oil. Opt for cold-pressed virgin oil; the quality justifies the expense.

As with all other oils, if you can find an organic option, it is an added bonus.

Peach-kernel oil

Very similar to apricot kernel oil in weight and appearance, peach kernel oil is also equally good for facial use.

Peanut (arachis) oil

Peanut oil is an oil that is very rich in minerals and vitamins. Some people with nut allergies suffer violent reactions to peanut oil, however. **Warning:** Always make sure that the subject is not allergic to nuts.

Sunflower oil

Sunflower oil contains vitamins A, B, D and E and is a cheaper option than some for use as a base oil. Be careful to look for cold-pressed sunflower oil, rather than picking up any old bottle of cooking oil from the supermarket. If it is organically produced, so much the better.

Wheatgerm oil

Wheatgerm oil is thick, rich and golden, and it is particularly rich in vitamin E – even more so then avocado oil. The vitamin E content helps to preserve the essential

oils that are added to it. It is best used in dilution with
another base oil, in a proportion of one to ten, as it is
heavy and viscous. **Warning:** Use with care on those
who are sensitive to or allergic to wheat – test on a
small patch of skin and wait for twenty-four hours to
check for any possible adverse reaction.

Macerated oils

Macerated or infused oils are base oils to which herbs
have been added. The herbs are left in the oil over a
period of time to allow their properties to infuse the base
oil thoroughly before being removed. These oils can also
be used as bases or carriers for the addition of essential
oils and have additional individual properties imparted by
the herbs that have been added to them. Macerated oils
include calendula oil (soothing), carrot oil (anti-inflammatory), and comfrey oil (healing).

Diluting essential oils for massage

Twenty drops essential oil = 1ml
1 tablespoon = 15ml
1 teaspoonful = 5ml

Dilution quantities of essential oil to base oil

For a 1 per cent dilution: 3 drops per tablespoonful/1 drop per teaspoonful

For a 2 per cent dilution: 6 drops per tablespoonful/2 drops per teaspoonful

For a 3 per cent dilution: 9 drops per tablespoonful/3 drops per teaspoonful

A–Z of Plants and their Essential Oils

CAUTION

Some essential oils are unsuitable for use at home and some medical conditions contra-indicate the use of certain essential oils and/or massage itself. Read the information that follows with care. If you want to enjoy the benefits of aromatherapy in your own home, please do so safely, paying attention to the contra-indications that are given. Aromatherapy oils can be used by an untrained person quite safely to aid relaxation, relieve stress and treat minor aches and pains, but treatment of all other complaints should be left to the experts.

If you are currently undergoing medical treatment for any condition or using another complementary therapy such as homeopathy or herbal medicine, seek the advice of the relevant practitioner as well as that of an aromatherapist. This will ensure that any aromatherapy treatment is working with the other therapy most effectively. You will also be able to ensure that there are no contra-indications for massage or the use of certain essential oils in your particular circumstances.

Be sure that you only use oils that are safe to use and use them in the appropriate manner. If you have any doubts about using essential oils or massage, seek the advice of a qualified aromatherapist. If you have a serious or chronic medical problem, consult a doctor before considering treatment with aromatherapy. Do not make any attempt to self-diagnose. If you suffer from a skin disorder or have a very sensitive skin, seek qualified advice before considering the use of essential oils. Pregnant women should avoid the use of essential oils in massage unless they have absolute, authoritative information about which oils are safe for them to use and how they should be used.

ANGELICA – *Angelica archangelica/ Angelica officinalis*

The plant
Angelica belongs to the family *Apiaceae* (*Umbelliferae*), the plant family to which fennel, dill and parsley also

belong. The plant is indigenous to Europe and is cultivated for commercial purposes in Germany, Belgium and
Hungary. It is a tall biennial, growing to a height of around
6–7 feet (1.8–2 metres).

Angelica has been used in herbal medicine for hundreds of years. In China it is used for gynaecological
problems and in Europe it is appreciated particularly for
its value in the treatment of urinary and respiratory disorders.

The candied stalks of the plant are commonly used in
cakes and confections, particularly in France, Italy and
Spain.

The oil
Essential oil of angelica is produced by the steam distillation of the roots or of the seeds.

The oil is colourless or pale yellow and has a strong
earthy, spicy fragrance. It is used for its fragrance in
the production of perfumes, soaps and cosmetics. It is
employed by the food and drinks industries as a
flavouring ingredient.

Therapeutically, angelica oil can be used in a variety of
ways. It has a strengthening effect on the spirits and can
also be used to treat nervous tension, anxiety and stress.

It will give a boost to the flagging mind and body when fatigue has set in, particularly if this is stress-induced. Use in massage blends or bathing for this purpose.

Angelica can also benefit the digestive system, combating indigestion and flatulence and boosting a jaded appetite.

The effects of the oil on the circulatory system are primarily stimulating and detoxifying. Angelica also has a diuretic effect so can be used to combat fluid retention.

Angelica has expectorant properties so can be used to treat catarrhal coughs. It will also help to reduce the feverishness that is associated with coughs, colds and influenza.

Used in skin care, angelica oil is particularly good for treating dull, lifeless skin and will also benefit dermatitis and psoriasis, soothing associated irritation.

Suitable methods of use
Bathing, inhalation, massage, skin care, vaporiser/diffuser

Precautions
Warning: Avoid during pregnancy. Not suitable for use by diabetics. Avoid exposure to the sun – may be phototoxic. Otherwise, generally safe to use.

ANISEED – *Pimpinella anisum*

The plant

Aniseed is a member of the *Umbelliferae* plant family, which includes several other commonly used herbs such as angelica, dill and fennel. The plant is native to the warmer climes of Egypt and Greece, and is now also grown in several other countries, including Spain and Mexico. The seeds of the plant have a pleasant liquorice taste and, as a result, aniseed is used in the confectionery industry and also as a flavouring for throat lozenges and cough preparations. Alcoholic beverages such as Pastis and Pernod are aniseed-flavoured and aniseed can be used as an ingredient in some recipes for home cooking.

Like fennel and dill, aniseed can have beneficial effects on the digestive system, combating flatulence, indigestion and colic. Aniseed also has a deodorising effect on the breath so is used in breath-freshening preparations. Other properties of the plant have enabled it to be used since the times of the ancient Romans as an aphrodisiac, an antiseptic and a stimulant to the production of breast milk in nursing mothers. Aniseed also has a decongestant effect on the upper respiratory tract.

The oil

The essential oil is obtained from the seed by steam distillation. The oil is very pale yellow in colour and has a sweet and spicy smell. It is used extensively in the pharmaceutical and food and drinks industries.

Aniseed oil is used therapeutically in the treatment of respiratory and digestive problems but has a relatively high level of toxicity. Although the plant and seeds have culinary and medicinal uses, the essential oil is not recommended for domestic use.

Precautions

Can cause drowsiness and dizziness in large doses and is an irritant, causing skin problems such as dermatitis in some people. **Warning:** Not recommended for use in the home, unless on the advice of a trained therapist.

BASIL (SWEET) – *Omicum basilicum*

The plant

Basil belongs to the *Lamiaceae* (*Labiatae*) family of plants. The aromatic leaves and stems of the plant are a mainstay of many dishes in European cookery, adding a fresh, distinctively pungent taste to salads and sauces. Although basil originally comes from Africa, the plant is relatively easy to grow, flourishing in the area around the Mediterranean in particular. Even in the cooler temperatures of Great Britain it is a popular annual herb to grow, either in warm, sheltered gardens or in pots on the windowsill. There are several different varieties of the plant: French basil is the variety used in aromatherapy. Much of the basil that is grown for essential oil production comes from Egypt.

Whilst all cooks will be well aware of the versatility of basil as a cooking ingredient, not all of them will know of the beneficial properties of the plant when it is eaten. It is effective as an antispasmodic agent and thus its consumption is a particularly pleasant way to aid digestion. Basil has been used in herbal medicine for hundreds of years for the treatment of fever and stomach and digestive complaints.

The oil

The whole plant is used for extracting the essential oil of basil, which is obtained by steam distillation. The oil is either colourless or pale yellow and has a sweet, spicy herbal smell. Basil oil is used as a fragrance ingredient in the cosmetics industry and is also used extensively in food production.

Basil oil has many therapeutic effects. It is both soothing and uplifting when diluted in a base oil and used for massage; it has the effect of relieving gloom and fatigue, generally lifting the spirits and promoting a sense of wellbeing. Massage with a blend containing basil oil can thus be a wonderful tonic for stress at the end of a hard working day and will also improve circulatory function. Bath oils containing essential oil of basil can make a soak in a warm tub all the more beneficial as inhalation and absorption of the oil both work their magic. Steam inhalation of the oil is a favoured treatment for many respiratory ailments, and basil is also known to be effective in soothing fever.

Basil oil will bring relief to insect bites and stings, applied in dilution, and also acts as an insect repellent.

Suitable methods of use
Bathing, inhalation, massage, vaporiser/diffuser.

Precautions
Avoid using neat. Dilute well to avoid skin irritation. Use

with moderation. **Warning:** Pregnant women should avoid the use of basil oil.

BAY – *Laurus nobilis*

The tree

The plant family to which bay belongs is *Lauraceae*, the same family as camphor and cinnamon. The essential oil is extracted by steam distillation of the dried leaves and berries of the bay plant.

Bay, or sweet bay as it is also known, originally comes from the area around the Mediterranean, but is quite easily grown in sheltered, sunny positions in this country. The tree grows to as much as 60 feet high (18 metres) and is evergreen.

Bay leaves are a common addition to stews and casseroles, whether fresh or dried, and bay is one of the standard ingredients of a classic bouquet garni. The leaves are used whole and are removed from the dish once cooking is complete and their flavour has infused throughout.

In common with most of the herbs that are widely used in cooking, bay has beneficial effects on the digestive system. Bay can also help to combat flatulence, and chewing on a bay leaf will help to freshen the breath after a spicy meal.

History reveals that bay was widely used in ancient Rome and Greece. Apart from its benefits as a digestive aid, it was believed to offer protection from malign spiritual influences. The emperors of ancient Rome wore wreaths of laurel (another name for bay) in time of victory and it remains a symbol of victory, wealth and importance to this day.

The oil

The essential oil is extracted from bay by steam distillation of the dried leaves and twigs. The oil is yellow-green in colour and smells strongly medicinal. Bay oil is used for its fragrance by the cosmetics and perfume industries and is also used in the production of a variety of foods and drinks.

Bay oil can be used in massage, bathing and inhalation. It has an uplifting effect on the spirits, and medicinally it can help in the treatment of minor respiratory illnesses such as colds and influenza. It helps combat flatulence and indigestion and can stimulate a jaded appetite. Bay oil is an emmenagogue – it can induce menstruation – and can help when periods are scanty and irregular.

Suitable methods of use
Massage (well-diluted), hair care, inhalation, vaporiser/diffuser.

Precautions
Bay oil can be irritating to sensitive skins. Use in proper dilution and in moderation only. Those with particularly sensitive or allergy-prone skins should avoid the use of bay oil in massage at home. **Warning:** Bay should not be used during pregnancy.

BENZOIN – *Styrax benzoin*

The plant
Benzoin is the resin obtained from the tree known as *Styrax benzoin*, a relative of *Styrax japonicus*, or the snowbell tree, belonging to the family *Styraceae*. The tree is native to Borneo, Malaya and Java. It grows to heights of more than 50 feet (15 metres).

Benzoin in its crude form is a resin collected from

the cut trunk of the tree. It is used in the East for its fragrance – primarily as an ingredient in incense – and also medicinally for infections of the urinary tract.

The oil

Benzoin, also known as gum bejamin, is an important ingredient in friar's balsam, or compound tincture of benzoin, which has been favoured for many years in the treatment of chesty colds and bronchitis. The essential oil – or resinoid – is produced from the resin by solvent extraction and is very viscous. Some kinds are solid. It is orange-amber in colour. It is generally sold in solution. Benzoin can be used to benefit the respiratory system by steam inhalation, is an effective expectorant and has an anti-inflammatory action that soothes laryngitis. Additionally its antiseptic properties can help in the treatment of throat and respiratory infections. Its vanilla-like fragrance makes it enjoyable to use.

In massage, mixed with a base oil, benzoin is used as a stress-reliever, relaxant and mood enhancer. It is invaluable in soothing 'jangled' nerves and will warm body and mind, do much to relieve rheumatic and arthritic pain and stimulate a sluggish circulation.

Benzoin is generally kind to the skin and can be used as a cleanser and as a treatment for dry and chapped skin. It is also used extensively in the cosmetics industry as a fragrant addition to the ingredients in bath products, shampoos and perfumes.

Suitable methods of use
Bathing, inhalation, massage, skin care, vaporiser/diffuser.

Precautions
Friar's balsam, or compound tincture of benzoin as it is also called, can be irritating to very sensitive skins, but any irritation is likely to be caused by the other components in the tincture rather than the benzoin itself, which is unlikely to cause problems of this nature. However, there can be problems with sensitisation to benzoin in a very small minority of people.

BERGAMOT – *Citrus bergamia*

The plant
Bergamot is an evergreen citrus fruit tree, a member of the family *Rutaceae*, which also includes citron, lemon,

lime, orange and tangerine. The fruit is also known as sweet orange and is distinctively pear-shaped. It originates from Asia and can be grown only in warm climates because the plant is not tolerant of frost.

The oil

The oil has a sharp and pungent fruity fragrance and is easily extracted, from the rind of the fruit in particular, by squeezing the rind in the process known as expression. This is done mechanically nowadays, although originally it was done by hand.

Oil of bergamot has been used for its therapeutic properties for many centuries in Europe. In Italy in particular it has been used to treat fever and worms. It is also a fragrant and flavoursome addition to many food products – Earl Grey tea, for example – and an important component of many perfumes and scented products, in particular, classic eau de Cologne.

Bergamot oil is a powerful antiseptic. In appropriate dilution, it has prove its use in the treatment of many troublesome skin complaints, such as eczema, some of which can be reluctant to respond to other forms of treatment. Stress-related complaints such as headaches and irritability will often respond well to a massage with oil of bergamot in the blend. The effect of the oil is vitalising and uplifting, soothing tension away without any sedative effect. The pleasant fragrance makes a lovely addition to a blend for a vaporiser.

Bergamot eases problem gastrointestinal spasm and flatulence and gentle abdominal massage can bring relief from constipation and colic. The oil is also detoxifying and is thought to help in the treatment of cellulite when used in massage. In addition to this, when used for bathing, bergamot oil can soothe inflammation and can help alleviate vaginal itching and the symptoms of cystitis. In inhalation or massage, it can be used in the treatment of respiratory infections such as sore throats and bronchitis. Bergamot can also be used in a mouthwash to deodorise bad breath and fight mouth and throat infections, or on the hair to control dandruff.

Suitable methods of use
Bathing, hair care, inhalation, massage, mouthwash, skin care, vaporiser/diffuser.

Precautions
Bergamot oil should not be used on the skin prior to exposure to the sun – it is phototoxic and can cause pig-

mentation. If possible, try to use bergapten-free oil which reliable suppliers of essential oils should stock.

BLACK PEPPER – *Piper nigrum*

The plant
Black pepper is the dried seed of the plant, a vine-like climber that belongs to the *Piperaceae* family and is grown for commercial purposes mainly in India and Indonesia. Its use as a spice goes back at least four thousand years and few cooks can do without it in their kitchen. Black pepper is highly regarded in Chinese medicine, particularly for the treatment of digestive disorders.

The oil
Black-pepper oil is extracted by steam distillation of the crushed, dried peppercorns. The oil is usually colourless, sometimes with a greenish or light amber tinge, and has a warm, freshly spicy smell. Black-pepper oil is used extensively by the food and drinks industry and is also employed in the manufacture of some perfumed products.

Black pepper is a warming oil and can be particularly beneficial in the treatment of heavy colds, when the patient feels shivery, achy, listless and depressed. It is both stimulating and energising. It can be used in massage or in a vaporiser. Used in massage, it will be of particular benefit to athletes and those with arthritic or rheumatic pain, poor circulation or chilblains, and it is comforting and warming in a footbath. Avoid using it in general bathing, as it can be irritating to the skin.

Suitable methods of use
Footbath, inhalation, massage.

Precautions
Use well diluted and in small amounts as it can be a skin irritant.

CAJEPUT – *Melaleuca cajeputi*

The plant
Cajeput, also known as white tea tree and related to tea tree, belongs to the plant family *Myrtaceae* and grows in Australia, Indonesia, Malaysia and Southeast Asia.

Cajeput is a very tall evergreen tree with whitish bark and white flowers. It is a commonly used plant in herbal medicine, in East and West alike, for the treatment of fever, respiratory and skin complaints.

The oil

The essential oil is obtained by the process of steam distillation from the leaves and twigs of the plant. It is pale greenish yellow in colour and smells fresh, herbal and medicinal. The oil is used extensively by the pharmaceutical industry and also in dentistry. It is an ingredient in cosmetics, detergents and cough and cold preparations.

Cajeput oil is quite an effective analgesic and can be used in the treatment of toothache when applied in a warm compress to the affected side of the face. Compresses can also be used to soothe the pain of strained muscles and bruises.

In skin care, cajeput can be used to treat insect bites if used in dilution. It can also help oily skin and acne.

Cajeput oil used in inhalation or massage can be particularly beneficial to the respiratory system. It is an expectorant and an antiseptic, and it will also be comfortingly warming to those who are suffering from colds and chills. The oil is one of the principal ingredients in Olbas oil, widely sold as a cold treatment.

In bathing, it also helps in the treatment of cystitis.

Suitable methods of use
Bathing (use very well diluted), compress, inhalation, massage, vaporiser/diffuser.

Precautions
Use well diluted and in moderation to avoid skin irritation. **Warning:** It is recommended that cajeput is avoided during the first three months of pregnancy.

CARDAMOM – *Elettaria cardamomum*

The plant
Cardamom belongs to the family *Zingiberaceae* and originates in India. It is a striking, large-leafed plant, growing to about 10 feet (3 metres) in height. The seeds of the plant have been used in Indian cookery for hundreds of years and are equally popular in many of the kitchens of the Western world. The essential oil gives the spice its distinctive warming, invigorating qualities. Chewing the

seeds can help to alleviate indigestion and heartburn and stimulate the digestive system into working more effectively. Much of the cardamom oil that is produced commercially comes from Guatemala.

The oil

Cardamom oil is extracted from the dried seeds of the plant by the process of steam distillation. It is either colourless or pale yellow and smells sweet, warm and spicy. It can be used in baths, massage or in vaporisers and its effect is warming, uplifting, invigorating to the spirits and imparting a sense of contentment to those who have been suffering from anxiety and stress. Cardamom oil is also believed to be an aphrodisiac and can be used in massage to stimulate a jaded sexual appetite.

Cardamom oil also benefits the digestive system, having a carminative (antiflatulent) and antispasmodic effect when mixed with a base oil and massaged gently over the abdomen. It can also be used in mouthwashes as it has antiseptic properties.

Suitable methods of use

Bathing, inhalation, massage, mouthwash, vaporiser/diffuser.

Precautions
Cardamom is generally non-toxic and non-irritant, but may cause skin irritation in some cases.

CARROT – *Daucus carota*

The plant
The carrot plant, a member of the *Umbelliferae* family, needs little introduction. A bright orange-red root vegetable with distinctive, feathery leaves, it is easy to grow, cheap to buy, a staple vegetable in the kitchen and rich in vitamins, particularly vitamins A and C. It is the seed of the wild carrot, a different variety of plant, from which the essential oil is extracted.

Carrot seeds are used in herbal medicine for kidney and bladder problems and also for some digestive disorders.

The oil
Carrot-seed oil is obtained by the process of steam distillation, after the seeds have been crushed. It is a golden oil with a warm, earthy smell. Carrot-seed oil has a variety of uses commercially as both a flavouring and perfuming ingredient in food and cosmetic products. It is used in

aromatherapy primarily in skin care preparations, puri-fying and revitalising tired and jaded complexions, tautening sagging skin and helping to heal pimples.

It can also be used in bathing and massage, its benefits being mainly to the skin but also relieving gout, arthritis and rheumatism. It can also help in the treatment of scanty periods.

Suitable methods of use
Bathing, massage, skin care, steam inhalation, vaporiser/diffuser

Precautions
None – carrot-seed oil is non-irritant and non-sensitising.

CEDARWOOD – *Cedrus atlantica*

The tree
Cedar originates from the Atlas mountains and is grown in particular in Morocco, from where most of the essential oil for aromatherapy is imported. Cedar belongs to the family *Pinaceae*. The trees are large and imposing. Demand for cedarwood for building and

furnishing has greatly depleted the ancient cedar forests of Lebanon, which is why the oil has to be sourced elsewhere. Another kind of cedarwood oil comes from the red cedar – *Juniperus virginiana* – which is grown in North America. Cedarwood itself is highly aromatic.

The oil

Cedarwood oil has a rich, honey colour and a warm, woody, sweet smell that appeals to both sexes. The oil is extracted from wood waste – sawdust, chips and shavings – by the process of steam distillation.

Cedarwood oil has been in use for many centuries. The ancient Egyptians used it in cosmetics and in the process of mummification. It is also used in incense. Nowadays, it is used commercially for its fragrance in a variety of household products and also in the manufacture of cosmetics and toiletries, in particular aftershaves. Aromatherapists use cedarwood oil for the treatment of respiratory ailments. It has antiseptic properties, and is effective against coughs, bronchitis and catarrh. Its use in skin and hair care is well recognised, and it can be very beneficial in the treatment of dandruff, eczema and acne. As an ingredient in a blend to perfume a room, cedarwood oil is warm and pleasant. The oil is particularly useful in treating stress and tension.

Suitable methods of use

Bathing, compresses, inhalation, massage, skin care, vaporiser/diffuser.

Precautions

Use in low concentration only as it can be irritating to the skin. **Warning:** Cedarwood oil must be avoided during pregnancy.

CHAMOMILE – *Anthemis nobilis/Matricaria chamomilla*

The plant

Both the above varieties of chamomile are used in aromatherapy. *Anthemis nobilis* is known as Roman chamomile, a low-growing herb with yellow, daisy-shaped heads that makes a soft and fragrant lawn when planted close together. Roman chamomile is perennial, but German chamomile – *Matricaria chamomilla* – is an annual herb and grows wild in, amongst other places, both Germany and Great Britain. Chamomile belongs to the plant family *Asteraceae* (*Compositae*).

Chamomile has been well regarded in herbal medicine for many centuries. It is calming in effect and is useful in treating nervous tension and insomnia. The herb is also used for hair and skin care. Chamomile tea, made from an infusion of the flower heads, is a refreshing and soothing drink, good for the digestion and an aid to a restful night's sleep.

The oil

Chamomile oil is blue in colour and has many benefits, particularly in skin care. It is widely used in the cosmetics industry in soaps, creams and shampoos. Chamomile is known to enhance and brighten the colour of blonde hair.

In aromatherapy, the uses of chamomile oil are many. It is soothing and relaxing, and when used for bathing can alleviate stress and anxiety, soothe menstrual cramps and relieve tension headaches. It will also do much to relieve vaginal irritation and itching. In massage its effects are equally calming and can do much to relieve muscle and joint pain and to promote relaxation in those of a fretful or irritable disposition. Chamomile is invaluable in the treatment of skin complaints such as allergies, eczema and pruritis. Its action is anti-inflammatory and antiseptic. It has analgesic properties and is useful in the treatment of earache and migraine. In compresses, chamomile oil will help relieve painful breasts, especially in the early days of breastfeeding.

Suitable methods of use
Bathing, compresses, hair care, inhalation, massage, skin care vaporiser/diffuser.

Precautions
Chamomile is safe to use in most circumstances, nontoxic and nonirritant, although it can cause skin irritation in those who are particularly sensitive. **Warning:** Some therapists recommend that chamomile is avoided during the first three months of pregnancy.

CINNAMON LEAF – *Cinnamomum zeylanicum*

The tree
Like bay, cinnamon belongs to the family *Lauraceae*. The trees, native to Sri Lanka but now found in many

other countries such as Brazil and Madagascar, are around 40 feet (12 metres) tall when they reach maturity. Cinnamon is a spice of age-old use. The trees are cultivated to form several stems at a time, and when the bark of the young twigs turns brown, the stems are cut. Cinnamon 'sticks', familiar to most cooks, are made from the inner and outer bark of these stems dried and rolled together. Cinnamon is a favoured ingredient in cookery both in the East and in the West. Its sweet, spicy taste makes it suitable for baking and puddings as well as for savoury dishes. Medicinally, cinnamon has a long history in Eastern medicine where it is used to treat fever and menstrual problems among other things.

The oil
There are two different oils extracted from the tree. Cinnamon-leaf oil has some use in aromatherapy, but cinnamon-bark oil is a strong irritant, high in toxicity and should not be used. Cinnamon-leaf oil is extracted from the leaves and young twigs of the tree by steam distillation. Commercially, it is used in the food and drinks industry in some sweets and carbonated drinks, and in the pharmaceutical industry it is used in cough medications and dental preparations.

Aromatherapists can use cinnamon-leaf oil in massage to relieve rheumatism, and it can also be beneficial in the treatment of digestive disorders. It is a stimulant and is used to treat circulatory problems. It can also be of benefit to those who are suffering from nervous exhaustion.

Suitable methods of use
Massage (well diluted), vaporiser/diffuser.

Precautions
Cinnamon-leaf oil is a skin irritant. Use very well diluted and in moderation. **Warning:** Do not confuse cinnamon-leaf oil with cinnamon-bark oil, which is unsuitable for aromatherapy.

CITRONELLA – *Cymbopogon nardus*

The plant
Citronella is native to and cultivated in Sri Lanka, particularly in the south of the island. Another variety of citronella, which is grown in Java, Vietnam, South and Central America – *Cymbopogon winterianus* – is also

used to produce oil. Citronella belongs to the plant family *Poaceae* (*Gramineae*)

Citronella is a perennial grass with aromatic leaves. The plant has a long history of use in the traditional herbal medicine of the countries in which it grows for the treatment of digestive problems and intestinal parasites and to combat fever. It is also used as an insect repellent.

The oil

Essential oil of citronella is produced by the process of steam distillation from the leaves – either fresh, partially dried or dried. The oil is yellow in colour and smells fresh and lemony.

Essential oil of citronella is used in the manufacture of some proprietary insect repellents. It is also used in household cleaning products and soaps.

Citronella is used primarily for skin care in aromatherapy. It is antiseptic and bactericidal and can be used to treat oily skin that is prone to spots. The oil is also useful as a deodoriser.

Citronella is a very effective insect repellent when well diluted in a carrier oil and applied to the skin. It can also be used in a vaporiser to deter insects from entering a room. It is an extremely useful oil to have in the home for this reason, especially in the summer months. Some gardeners use citronella to stop cats from digging around plants in the garden.

Used in a compress, citronella can help relieve headaches and migraine. The effect of the oil is uplifting and can help to cheer the spirits.

Suitable methods of use
Massage (dilute well), skin care, vaporiser/diffuser.

Precautions
Warning: Avoid during pregnancy (citronella is an emmenagogue). Can cause skin irritation, so always dilute well.

CLARY SAGE – *Salvia sclarea*

The plant
Clary sage belongs to the family *Lamiaceae* (*Labiatae*). It originally comes from Syria, but has been growing in Britain since the sixteenth century. It is an elegant plant with hairy leaves, growing to approximately 3 feet (0.9 metres) in height. It is grown in several

countries now, and is cultivated on a commercial basis in Spain and France.

It has been used medicinally since the Middle Ages for many ailments, in particular eye disease – 'clary' may be derived from 'clear eye'.

Clary sage is safer to use than garden (common) sage and is therefore the plant of choice for aromatherapy. Common sage oil has a high level of toxicity and is unsuitable for therapeutic use.

The oil

Both leaves and flowers are used to obtain the essential oil of clary sage, the oil being extracted by the process of steam distillation. The oil has a distinctively herbal smell, light and quite sweet – almost flowery – with an edge that gives it a hint of bitterness. It is pale yellow in colour. Clary-sage oil is used by perfumers in France as a fixative for many perfumes and it is also used in the production of some foods and drinks.

Clary-sage oil can be used to treat a variety of problems. It has a sedating effect, calming tension and creating a feeling of greater wellbeing, while at the same time lifting the mood. It will be of use to anyone who feels weak and debilitated after illness, cheering flattened spirits and provoking feelings of optimism, and it is recommended for use in vaporisers or diffusers anywhere creative people are working as its effects are considered to be quite inspirational. Some people report that they have had particularly vivid dreams after using the oil. Used in large quantities, however, clary sage can cause drowsiness. Alcohol should be avoided if using the oil because the combination of the two can produce a strongly narcotic effect.

Clary sage is useful in the treatment of menstrual cramping – gentle abdominal massage or the application of warm compresses is recommended – and massage or bathing with clary sage can be of benefit to women who are feeling particularly low after childbirth, suffering from premenstrual tension or going through the menopause. Its antispasmodic properties can be helpful to both the digestive and the respiratory system, and when used for the treatment of stress it has the added advantage of being anti-hypertensive.

When used in inhalation, clary sage is beneficial to those suffering from colds or bronchitis; it is anti-inflammatory, antiseptic and helps in the healing process. The oil has astringent, toning, bactericidal and antiseptic properties that make it good for treating greasy skin.

Suitable methods of use
Bathing, compresses, inhalation, massage, skin care, vaporiser/diffuser.

Precautions
Warning: Avoid during pregnancy. Use in moderation. Avoid consuming alcohol if using clary sage. Avoid driving immediately after treatment. Not to be confused with common sage – *Salvia officinalis* – which is unsafe to use.

CLOVE – *Eugenia aromatica*

The tree
The clove tree is native to Indonesia but now grows in several countries. The tree is evergreen and of small to medium size. It belongs to the family *Myrtaceae*. Cloves, as we are familiar with them, are the flower buds of the tree, not yet open, which have been dried in wood smoke. Cloves have been a common flavouring ingredient in the cookery of several countries for many years and the deodorising, antiseptic and anaesthetic properties of the essential oil have been appreciated by

different cultures, in particular the Chinese, for centuries.

The oil
Oil of cloves is obtained by the process of water distillation from the buds of the tree. Essential oils are also obtained from the twigs and leaves of the tree, but these are more toxic than the bud oil and are to be avoided.

The powerful anaesthetic properties of clove oil ensure that it is a staple in the dentist's surgery. Dressings containing clove oil are very effective in cleansing and soothing holes in the teeth and aching empty tooth sockets. Some toothpastes also contain oil of cloves. For the treatment of toothache at home, put a drop of clove oil in a tablespoonful of warm water, soak some cotton wool in this, screw up a tiny ball of the cotton wool and apply this to the affected tooth; relief will be instantaneous, even if the taste is distinctly 'nippy'. Do not swallow. A safer alternative is to use tincture of cloves, which contains clove oil but is less concentrated and is available from most good pharmacies.

Clove oil can also be used by aromatherapists in massage for the treatment of certain fungal skin conditions and catarrh and bronchitis but is not advised for home use.

Precautions
Clove oil has a relatively high level of toxicity so it is recommended that you restrict its use at home to emergency dental analgesia. **Warning:** Clove oil is recommended to be used only by trained therapists.

CORIANDER – *Coriandrum sativum*

The plant
Coriander is believed to be indigenous to Asia and southern Europe but is now grown extensively throughout Europe and North America. The oil is produced in various countries, including Russia and Romania.

Coriander, a member of the plant family *Apiaceae* (*Umbelliferae*), is an annual herb, approximately 3 feet (0.9 metres) high with delicate, fragrant leaves, resembling those of parsley, and green, spherical, highly aromatic seeds produced in abundance. The leaves are used extensively in cookery and have a pleasantly fresh taste, almost orange-like. The seeds, either fresh or dried, are also popular in cooking and are an ingredient in many curry dishes.

Coriander has been used since ancient times. The tomb of the Egyptian Pharaoh Rameses II was found to contain coriander seeds. Coriander has been used in herbal medicine for the treatment of digestive complaints both in China and in Western countries.

The oil

Essential oil of coriander is obtained from the seeds, when ripe, by steam distillation. The oil is colourless or very pale yellow and has a fresh, sweet, spicy odour. Coriander oil is used in the pharmaceutical industry as a flavouring ingredient. It is also used in the manufacture of cosmetics, soaps and some perfumes. The food industry utilises coriander oil as a flavouring agent.

Therapeutically, coriander is warming and stimulating on the nervous and circulatory systems. It is comforting and revitalising and will help to boost confidence and combat debility when spirits are low. It is also beneficial in the treatment of muscular stiffness and aches and pains associated with rheumatism and arthritis. It has analgesic properties and will warm and soothe areas of pain and discomfort.

Coriander oil can be used to alleviate some of the symptoms of digestive problems, particularly when used in massage. It has antispasmodic properties and will relieve flatulence, colic and dyspepsia. It can help to stimulate a poor appetite, especially after illness. It can also help in the treatment of diarrhoea.

Coriander is useful in the treatment of post-illness weakness and 'blues'. It also has aphrodisiac properties and can stimulate a jaded sexual appetite when used in massage or in bathing.

The fragrance blends well with spice oils for use in a vaporiser.

Suitable methods of use
Bathing, compresses, inhalation, massage, vaporiser/diffuser.

Precautions
Coriander is nontoxic and non-sensitising, and when used in dilution it will not irritate the skin. It can, however, have a stupefying effect if used in very large doses –

moderation is therefore advised. **Warning:** Avoid using coriander during pregnancy.

CUMIN – *Cuminum cyminum*

The plant
Cumin is an annual herb, a member of the plant family *Apiaceae* (*Umbelliferae*) to which several other aromatic herbs such as parsley, coriander and dill also belong. Cumin originally comes from Egypt but has been cultivated in India and in Mediterranean countries for centuries. The fragrant, flavoursome seeds of the plant are a spice ingredient in many Indian dishes, and cumin has also been used medicinally in India, particularly as a digestive aid. Cumin is cultivated commercially in India, France and Spain.

The oil
Essential oil of cumin is obtained by the process of steam distillation from the ripe seeds of the plant. The oil is yellow and smells warmly spicy. Oil of cumin is used as an ingredient in some perfumes and also as a fragrance component in various cosmetics. It is used in the food and drinks industry as a flavouring agent.

Therapeutically, cumin can be used to treat digestive disorders and help in the elimination of toxins. Cumin oil is beneficial in the treatment of sluggish circulation and/or fluid retention, particularly when used in massage. It can also be used to good effect to assist the digestive process. It is carminative and antispasmodic so will combat flatulence and colic and soothe the discomfort of indigestion.

Cumin oil has a stimulating effect on the nervous system and can help in the treatment of nervous fatigue and weakness. It can also help to relieve headaches, particularly if these are stress-induced.

Suitable methods of use
Bathing, inhalation, massage, vaporiser/diffuser

Precautions
Warning: Phototoxic – do not allow treated skin to be exposed to sunlight within twelve hours of application.

In other respects, cumin is safe to use. It is non-sensitising and non-irritant.

CYPRESS – *Cupressus sempervirens*

The tree

Cypress belongs to the *Cupressaceae* family of trees. This stately tree was believed to be sacred in ancient Greece and cypress branches were placed on the graves of the dead to facilitate their passage into the afterlife. Cypress trees originally came from the Eastern Mediterranean countries but can now be found throughout Europe. Cypress is often used as an ingredient in incense and is used in the cosmetics industry widely, its sweet, fresh, invigorating smell appealing to both sexes.

The oil

Cypress oil is extracted from the young twigs and needles of the tree by the process of steam distillation. It is pale yellowish green and smells sweet, fresh and woody.

The oil is very refreshing when used in the bath or in massage, a great comfort for rheumatism, aching limbs and stress-induced fatigue at the end of a long, hard day. Cypress oil in the bath will also benefit those who are suffering from haemorrhoids, bladder irritation or

111

the miseries of colds. Massage with cypress oil will help to relieve menorrhagia (excessive menstrual bleeding) and associated pelvic cramping. It will also help to stimulate the circulation. Its effects on the skin are primarily astringent and toning, and cypress has antiseptic properties. Used in facial massage, or in steam, it will benefit oily skin. It is soothing and deodorising in a footbath and in steam inhalation will benefit catarrhal coughs and bronchitis.

Cypress oil makes a pleasant addition to a vaporiser in a room, adding freshness and energy to the atmosphere. Its effects on the spirits are stimulating, uplifting and energising. It will also help to repel insects from the room.

Suitable methods of use

Bathing, compresses, inhalation, massage, skin care, vaporiser/diffuser/burner.

Precautions

None. Non-toxic non-sensitising and non-irritant if used in dilution.

DILL – *Anethum graveolens*

The plant

Dill comes from the same plant family as fennel – the *Apiacea* (*Umbelliferae*) – and both the herb and the oil have certain properties in common. Dill is native to Mediterranean countries but is now grown all over the world for use as a culinary and medicinal herb and for the production of its oil. The oil is produced in several countries, including France, Germany, Spain and England. Dill is a tall annual or biennial plant. It has feathery leaves and yellow flowers and produces copious quantities of small aromatic seeds. Both the seeds and the flowers are used extensively in cookery. The gentle flavour, like that of aniseed, makes a pleasing companion to fish dishes in particular. Dill has been appreciated as a digestive aid for a very long time and it is one of the ingredients of gripe water which is used to relieve colic in children.

The oil

Two oils are distilled from dill: one from the plant, either fresh or dried, and another from the seed. Essential oil of dill is used extensively in the food and drinks industries as a flavouring, particularly in alcoholic beverages and pickles. Dill oil is also used in the manufacture of various cosmetics, toiletries and cleaning products as a perfuming ingredient and has some uses in the pharmaceutical industry in addition to this.

Dill oil is primarily used for the benefit of the digestive system in aromatherapy. It is carminative and antispasmodic so, when used in massage in particular, will relieve uncomfortable and distressing flatulence and colic. It also acts as a general aid to digestion.

Dill oil, like fennel oil, can be used to help promote lactation in nursing mothers. It can also be used to treat amenorrhoea (absence of mensturation).

Used in a vaporiser, dill will combine successfully with a variety of other essential oils to give a room a pleasant fragrance.

Suitable methods of use
Bathing, inhalation, massage, vaporiser/diffuser.

Precautions
Dill oil is nontoxic, non-sensitising and generally nonirritant, although it may cause some irritation to those with very sensitive skins. **Warning:** Avoid use during pregnancy.

EUCALYPTUS – *Eucalyptus globulus*

The plant

Eucalyptus, a member of the family *Myrtaceae*, originally comes from Australia and Tasmania, but has been introduced to many other countries in the past two centuries, now being cultivated in Brazil, China, Spain, California and India among others. There are more than four hundred varieties of eucalyptus, but *Eucalyptus globulus*, or Tasmanian blue gum as it is also known, is the one from which the essential oil used in aromatherapy is extracted. Its history as a herb used in folk medicine stretches back several hundred years – the aboriginal people of Australia used it a great deal, particularly in the treatment of fever. The trees are highly aromatic, and it is wonderful to stand amongst them breathing in their aroma, especially after rain. Their presence in planting schemes near buildings helps to deter insects. In some places the trees are planted as a preventative measure against malaria, and anywhere where eucalyptus trees grow will benefit from the fragrance and the healthy atmosphere that they give to the area.

Eucalyptus is widely used by the pharmaceutical and confectionary industries. It is a component in various cough medicines, throat sweets, ointments, sports liniments and toothpaste.

The oil

Eucalyptus oil is one of the most popular and commonly used essential oils. It is obtained from the leaves of the tree by the process of steam extraction. The uses of eucalyptus oil are many. Few people will respond negatively to its stimulating, clean aroma. Its effects are warming, invigorating and refreshing, and it has strong antiseptic, anaesthetic and healing properties. It can be used in steam inhalations, baths and massage, and it is particularly beneficial in the treatment of respiratory infections such as bronchitis, croup and tracheitis. When used in vaporisers and spray diffusers it not only deodorises the atmosphere but also acts as a bactericidal fumigating agent. A vaporiser or a bowl of hot water, with a few drops of eucalyptus oil added, placed in the room of a person suffering from a stuffy nose or a troublesome cough, will do much to aid a restful night's sleep. A few drops of eucalyptus oil on a pillow will help to decongest a blocked nose and will be much appreciated by sufferers of sinusitis. During the day, a handkerchief to which eucalyptus oil has been applied can be used for inhalation purposes.

Used as an ingredient in massage oil, the warming effect of eucalyptus is therapeutic for muscular pain and stiffness.

A couple of drops of eucalyptus oil in a sitz bath will help in the treatment of urinary tract infections. The bactericidal and antiseptic properties of the oil also make it suitable for treatment of skin lesions, but it must be used in dilution as it is very strong and can irritate the skin. It can be used to treat athlete's foot, insect bites parasitic conditions such as ringworm and head lice, and it is soothing in the treatment of herpes and shingles.

Eucalyptus oil is an effective insect repellent, either used in a room spray or sprinkled on strips of ribbon hung from the ceiling (but keep these well away from light bulbs and heat sources).

Suitable methods of use
Bathing, compresses, inhalation, massage, vaporiser/diffuser.

Precautions
Eucalyptus oil is irritating to the skin. Always dilute well. Eucalyptus oil is potent and a little goes a long way. It does not have to be used in large quantities to

have the desired effect: three drops will suffice for a bath. Use sparingly in blends to avoid the fragrance overpowering others. Some therapists recommend that eucalyptus oil is not used in early pregnancy. **Warning:** Eucalyptus oil is very toxic if taken internally.

FENNEL (SWEET) – *Foeniculum vulgare (var. dulce)*

The plant
Fennel is a tall, graceful member of the *Umbelliferae* family and, although native to Mediterranean countries, grows freely throughout Europe. The plant is widely used in cookery, where its feathery leaves and celery-like stems impart a delicious flavour to many recipes. It tastes similar to aniseed. Fennel seed is an important ingredient in Indian cookery.

As with many of the herbs that are used in cookery, fennel has a beneficial, regulatory and balancing effect on the digestive system. It is antiflatulent, antispasmodic and gently laxative. Fennel tea is a popular digestive aid and anti-colic treatment. The herb is also thought to stimulate lactation in breastfeeding mothers.

The oil

Fennel oil is extracted by steam distillation from the seeds of the plant. It is very strong in odour, and in colour is clear with a slightly yellow tinge. It has bactericidal properties and is an ingredient in some toothpastes and mouthwashes, as it combats some of the bacteria that cause tooth decay.

Its antibacterial, laxative and carminative properties have made it popular with the pharmaceutical industry where it is used extensively. It is also an ingredient in some perfumed products.

Used in massage, particularly over the lower abdomen and back, fennel oil will soothe a nervous indigestion or irritated bowel. Flatulence and bloating can also be helped with gentle massage. Those who have problems with micturation often find that fennel helps to produce a steadier stream of urine. Its mild diuretic action can help with excessive fluid retention. Because of its strong odour, you may well find that fennel does not make a pleasing blend with other oils, but as its use tends to be more therapeutic than sensual, there is no need to blend fennel oil with other oils. Always dilute it well as it is strong and can irritate the skin – a 1° per cent dilution is quite sufficient.

Fennel can be used in vaporisers and because of its
expectorant qualities is thought to help catarrhal coughs
because of its expectorant qualities. Fennel has an effect
similar to that of the hormone oestrogen – this is why it
is used to stimulate lactation and increase milk production
– and it is not suitable for use during pregnancy.

Suitable methods of use
Compresses, inhalation, massage, mouthwashes, vapor-
iser/diffuser.

Precautions
Sweet fennel can cause sensitisation and should be well
diluted before use. **Warning:** Sweet fennel can be narcotic
if used in quantity. Do not use during pregnancy. Not to be
used on people suffering from epilepsy. Bitter fennel
(*Foeniculum vulgare var. amara*) should be avoided. It
is stronger and more likely to cause sensitisation.

FRANKINCENSE – *Boswellia carteri*

The tree
The tree from which frankincense resin is obtained grows

in Somalia, China and Ethiopia. It is a member of the family *Burseraceae*. Frankincense was greatly valued in ancient times by the Chinese, the Romans, the Egyptians and the Arabs for its rich aroma and for its stimulant properties. It is to this day an important part of religious and ceremonial proceedings throughout the world and is used in the preparation of incense.

The oil

The oil is extracted from the gum resin by the process of steam distillation. It is an ingredient in a wide variety of commercially produced perfumed products. It is clear in colour, with a tinge of pale yellow. Its smell is woody, sweet and warm with a strong element of pine. It blends well with many other oils. It is both soothing and uplifting when used in a burner or vaporiser. Many people use it as an aid to meditation as it can help slow down breathing and aid concentration, and it is an invaluable weapon in the war against stress.

Frankincense makes a good addition to a steam inhalation – its anti-inflammatory properties are useful in the treatment of bronchitis and laryngitis, and it will also help troublesome coughs by soothing irritated mucous membranes and assisting expectoration.

Cosmetically, frankincense is particularly valuable. Its action is astringent, antiseptic and toning. It is popular in the treatment of ageing skin.

Frankincense is a particularly safe and comforting essential oil to use.

Suitable methods of use
Bathing, compresses, inhalation, massage, skin care, vaporiser/diffuser.

Precautions
None. Non-toxic and non-irritant if used in dilution.
Warning: Some therapists recommend that frankincense is avoided during early pregnancy.

GARLIC – *Allium sativum*

The plant
Garlic, a member of the plant family *Liliacea*, is grown widely throughout Europe and is renowned for its antiseptic properties. The plant has been used over many centuries in different countries as a protection against evil. Garlic also has antibacterial and anti-hypertensive

properties and is greatly favoured as a flavouring ingredient in cookery worldwide, even if some people are intolerant of the effects that it has on the breath. There is no doubt that its consumption is beneficial to the health and if everybody ate it, the disadvantages of its smell on the breath – and in perspiration – would go unnoticed. Garlic capsules, which have all the advantages of large 'doses' of garlic but claim to be odour-free, are widely available in pharmacies and health food stores. Cooking with garlic and eating it, however gives much greater pleasure.

Because of its particular potency there is a little experiment you can perform using garlic that shows the effects of essential oils. Choose a day when you have not eaten garlic for some time. Peel and crush a garlic clove and rub it into the skin of your feet. Wait for an hour or so and then ask someone to smell your breath – remember, the essential oil would be much more concentrated in its effect than this!

The oil

Essential oil of garlic is a powerful antiseptic – possibly the most powerful among essential oils. It is unfortunate, therefore, that its overpowering smell makes its use virtually unbearable. It is just too strong and would never combine successfully with other oils. Aromatherapy is generally pleasant; the introduction of essential oil of garlic to an aromatherapist's repertoire would make both therapist and patient quite unpopular!

Precautions
Use of garlic oil renders all who touch it offensive to others. **Warning:** Not suitable for use at home.

GERANIUM – *Pelargonium graveolens*

The plant
Pelargonium graveolens, a member of the family *Geraniaceae*, originally comes from South Africa. It is also known as rose geranium and is grown now in countries as diverse as France, Egypt, North Africa and Russia. It is an attractive plant to look at and, like all members of the plant family to which it belongs, a pleasure to see in flower. The leaves are highly aromatic and give off a distinctive smell when brushed against or rubbed between the fingers. Varieties of geranium have been used since ancient times in the herbal medicine of different countries.

The oil

Geranium oil has been an important asset to the perfume industry ever since it was first distilled in France in the early eighteenth century. The essential oil is extracted by steam distillation from the leaves and stems of the plant, which are harvested just before flowering begins, when the scent of the plant is strongest. The oil is green in colour and smells fresh and rosy.

The properties of geranium oil are varied, but in the main it is an oil that is highly valued for its balancing, regulating qualities. It can be used in massage, bathing, or inhalation (either directly, in steam inhalation, or in a room vaporiser) and has the advantage of being generally nontoxic and nonirritant.

Geranium oil is often used in the treatment of menstrual disorders, especially premenstrual tension with associated fluid retention, and menopausal problems such as hot flushes. Its action is soothing and calming, and it works to alleviate anxiety and jumpiness, or restlessness, without having any unwanted sedative effect. It has analgesic and anti-inflammatory properties and, when used in the bath, will soothe the heat of acute cystitis and can also relieve some of the discomfort of chickenpox or the pain of shingles.

The anti-inflammatory properties of geranium oil also make it a favoured choice in the treatment of many skin conditions, such as eczema and acute dermatitis. It is also quite effective in the treatment of acne. Because of its balancing qualities, geranium oil can be used for the benefit of both dry and oily skins with no ill effects. In blends, geranium is one of the oils with a fragrance that blends well with many others, increasing its versatility.

Suitable methods of use
Bathing, compresses, hair care, inhalation, massage, skin care, vaporiser/diffuser.

Precautions
None. Geranium is generally perfectly safe to use in dilution on all but the most hypersensitive skins.

GINGER – *Zingiber officinale*

The plant
Ginger is native to Asia but is now grown widely throughout the tropics. The Caribbean countries, where the plant

has been grown for some four hundred years, depended on ginger as an important part of the spice trade. The ginger plant is a perennial herb with a tuberous rhizome, and this is the part of the plant that is used. The ginger flower is white or yellow and very showy. The spice turmeric, familiar to all those who are acquainted with Indian cookery, comes from another rhizome, *Curcuma longa*, which belongs to the same plant family, *Zingiberaceae*. An essential oil is also obtained from turmeric but it is an irritant and not safe for home use.

Ginger has a long history of use both as a spice and as a herbal remedy, in particular for ailments of a digestive nature. Its effects are stimulative and carminative, so relieving flatulence. Crystallised stem ginger is used in the manufacture of sweets and preserves. Ginger-based remedies can be used as a remedy for both travel sickness and the morning sickness of early pregnancy.

The oil

Essential oil of ginger is obtained from the root, which has been previously dried and ground, by the process of steam distillation. It is pale yellow to amber in colour and has a spicy, sweet and pungent smell.

Ginger oil is used as a fragrance ingredient in some

perfumes and is widely utilised in the food and drinks industry as a flavouring.

In aromatherapy, ginger can be used to help a variety of problems. The oil is warming and toning and can boost flagging spirits and strengthen resolve. When used in massage, ginger is particularly beneficial in the treatment of musculo-skeletal aches and pains that are more severe in cold, damp weather. It also helps to stimulate sluggish circulation and will work well on cold extremities. A footbath with ginger oil can be very soothing. Ginger oil can irritate the mucous membranes, however, and for this reason it is not recommended for use in full immersion baths.

Ginger oil, like the root of the plant, can be used to benefit the digestive system. It can be used to relieve nausea in the first three months of pregnancy and also travel-sickness. Inhalation from a handkerchief onto which one or two drops of ginger oil have been placed will bring relief. Ginger oil will stimulate a sluggish digestive system and will relieve associated flatulence. Use in massage blends or inhale for this purpose.

Ginger oil can also benefit the respiratory system, particularly if used in steam inhalation. It is an effective expectorant and so helps to clear the throat and nasal passages of excess mucus. It also does much to soothe an irritating cough and is thought to strengthen the body's immunity to the coughs and colds that winter brings. The oil will also help to reduce fever by encouraging sweating, which allows the body to cool down.

Ginger oil is an aphrodisiac.

Suitable methods of use
Compresses, footbaths (full immersion baths not recommended because of possible mucous membrane irritation), inhalation, massage, vaporiser/diffuser.

Precautions
Ginger is nontoxic and non-sensitising. It should be used with care as it can irritate mucous membranes but is suitable for use on the skin in appropriate dilution.

GRAPEFRUIT – *Citrus paradisi*

The plant
Grapefruit is one of the citrus fruits that has a sharper, almost bitter taste. It is grown in the United States, Caribbean countries, Spain and also in Israel. It is larger than the orange or lemon and generally has a yellow

skin. Pink grapefruit, less common but equally good, has a pink tinge to the skin and pink flesh. The taste of a grapefruit is such that it feels as if it is beneficial to the health, and it is. The sharp, fresh taste feels cleansing on the palate and wakes up the senses at the start of a day. Grapefruit is rich in vitamin C and is recommended as part of a detoxifying diet.

The oil
Essential oil of grapefruit is obtained from the skin and rind of the fruit by expression (machine pressing). The oil has a pleasant, fresh and sharp smell, much like the fruit, and is used by the cosmetic industry in many bath products, shampoos, soaps, etc.

The effects of grapefruit oil are primarily cooling, cleansing and detoxifying. A few drops of grapefruit oil in the bath act as a wonderful boost to flagging spirits. The bather will emerge feeling clean, fresh and new. In massage it can be used to help combat cellulite. Grapefruit is a valuable detoxifying agent and acts on the liver and kidneys to help the body to eliminate waste and toxins. It will play a useful part in any detoxifying regime, and some people recommend it as an aid to the process of drug withdrawal.

Grapefruit oil also helps in the digestive process, and gentle abdominal massage will help to relieve a sluggish digestion or constipation.

Used in inhalation or in vaporisers, grapefruit oil combines well with many others in a harmonious blend.

In skin preparations, the actions of grapefruit oil are cleansing and astringent, making it ideal for the treatment of excessive oiliness. It has a similar effect in hair treatments.

Suitable methods of use
Bathing, compresses, inhalation, massage, hair care, skin care, vaporiser/diffuser.

Precautions
Warning: Mildly phototoxic so avoid exposure to the sun after treatment. Dilute well.

HYSSOP – *Hyssopus officinalis*

The plant
Hyssop is a member of the plant family *Lamiaceae* (*Labiatae*). It is indigenous to Mediterranean countries

but now grows freely throughout Europe, in Russia and in the United States of America. It is cultivated for oil production in France, Italy, Spain, Hungary and the Balkan countries.

The plant is bushy and is a perennial. It grows to a height of approximately 5 feet (1.5 metres). It has small pointed leaves and flowers that vary in colour from pink, through violet to blue.

The herb has been used for many years in traditional herbal medicine, mainly for digestive ailments or problems of a respiratory nature, in particular coughs and bronchitis.

The oil
The essential oil of hyssop is obtained from the leaves and flowers of the plant by the process of steam distillation. The oil is colourless or pale greenish yellow and has a fragrance that is fresh and spicy. It is used for this fragrance in the production of soaps and other toiletries and also in the production of perfume. Hyssop oil is also employed in the manufacture of some food and drink products as a flavouring agent.

Therapeutically, hyssop has several possible applications, but it also has a certain amount of toxicity so should be used with care. Seek the advice of a trained therapist before using it at home. Hyssop oil is sedative in effect and can be used to treat anxiety, nervous tension and stress, either in bathing or in massage.

Hyssop is particularly beneficial in the treatment of respiratory ailments. It is antiseptic, antiviral and bactericidal and will help combat colds, influenza, bronchitis, asthma and sore throats. It also has expectorant properties that will help in the treatment of catarrh. It is antispasmodic so will soothe persistent irritating coughs.

Hyssop is an emmenagogue so can be used to treat amenorrhoea (absence of periods). Because of these properties it is unsuitable for use during pregnancy.

Hyssop can be used to regulate high or low blood pressure. Those who suffer from either problem should, however, seek qualified advice as it is important to find the cause in order to determine what treatment is appropriate.

In massage or in bathing, hyssop can also bring relief from flatulence and colic.

Hyssop can be used in skin care to soothe dermatitis and eczema.

Essential oil of hyssop should be used with care as it has a degree of toxicity.

Precautions

Warning: Not to be used during pregnancy. Has a degree of toxicity – use in strict moderation. Not to be used by epileptics. Not recommended for home use unless on the advice of a trained therapist.

JASMINE – *Jasminum officinale/ Jasminum grandiflorum*

The plant

Jasmine, a member of the plant family *Oleaceae*, originally comes from the northwest regions of India. It is an attractive climbing plant with delicate, pinkish-white flowers that exude a heady and delicious perfume. It is now cultivated for its oil in several countries, including Morocco, Egypt and France. Jasmine has been a mainstay of the perfume industry in France for many years now, in spite of the expense involved in the process of extracting its precious essential oil. The sensual qualities of jasmine have long been appreciated, as have its applications in skin care. It has also been used in the herbal medicine of East and West alike for the treatment of a variety of complaints.

The oil

Essential oil of jasmine is very expensive, simply because it is yielded in such small quantities. An astonishing amount of flowers is required to produce a small quantity of oil. The oil is extracted from the flowers of the plant, either by the process of enfleurage, a process still preferred by a very few perfume producers in spite of its labour intensiveness, or by solvent extraction. In spite of its expense, jasmine oil is highly esteemed in the perfume industry and is also an ingredient of many soaps, bath products, shampoos, etc. In addition, it is used to some extent by the food and drinks industry.

The oil is amber-brown in colour and quite viscous. Its odour is rich, sweet and strongly floral. Few people dislike the scent of jasmine, and it is widely appreciated for its powerful aphrodisiac qualities which affect both sexes. It is sometimes used as an ingredient of incense. Beware of cheap imitations!

Therapeutically, jasmine is valued for its antidepressant properties. Jasmine is useful in the treatment of emotional pain and stress-related depression. It induces a feeling of calm relaxation and can lift the spirits considerably. When used in massage, it will bring comfort to those who are sad or worn down by the burdens of life. It is beneficial during childbirth – diluted and massaged into the area of the lower back it will help to relieve pain and relax the mother-to-be. In sensual massage, jasmine will increase the pleasure of both partners, and it can be beneficial in the treatment of loss of libido or impotence, especially if this is stress-induced.

In skin care, jasmine is balancing and gentle. Its anti-inflammatory properties make it suitable for the treatment of irritated and inflamed skin in particular, but all skin types, dry and greasy alike, can benefit from jasmine.

Jasmine makes a delicious addition to a vaporiser in a room, giving it an air of cheerful calm, and it has also been recommended for helping to lift the spirits of new mothers who are suffering from fatigue and 'post-baby blues'. Jasmine combines successfully in many blends – the ease with which a harmonious blend can be created using jasmine oil adds to its versatility. The fragrance works particularly well in combination with citrus oils. The fragrance of jasmine oil is so powerful and long-lasting that, although it is costly, a little really does go a long way.

Suitable methods of use
Bathing, compresses, inhalation, massage, skin care, vaporiser/diffuser.

Precautions

Jasmine is generally nontoxic and nonirritant but can produce an allergic reaction in some extremely sensitive individuals.

JUNIPER – *Juniperus communis*

The tree

Juniper, an evergreen shrub/tree native to several countries in the Northern Hemisphere, belongs to the family *Cupressaceae*. The tree has needles that are bluish-green in colour and produces small, round black berries. The berries and needles of the juniper tree have a long history in traditional medicine and have been used to treat urinary disorders such as cystitis, various respiratory disorders, gout and rheumatism. It was also believed in medieval times to have magical properties against the black forces of witchcraft. Extracts of juniper are used in veterinary medicine for the treatment of parasitic infections. It is an ingredient in many perfumed products.

The berries of the juniper tree can be used in cookery and are also used in the process of making gin, giving the drink its distinctive perfume and flavour. Juniper is cultivated for commercial production of the essential oil in Italy and the Balkan countries.

The oil

Juniper oil is produced from the berries and also from the needles and twigs by the process of steam distillation. The oil is pale yellow in colour, and has a pleasingly fresh and woody, warm, sweet fragrance. It is a traditional component of incense and has many uses in aromatherapy. Its diuretic and antiseptic properties make it useful in the treatment of bladder disorders and fluid retention. It also helps in the elimination of toxins, in particular uric acid, making it useful in the treatment of gout. In massage it will also help rheumatic problems and menstrual disorders and is warming and stimulating.

Juniper is beneficial in the treatment of stress and anxiety as it has a calming effect on the emotions and will help promote positive feelings.

Juniper oil can be used in skin care for the treatment of greasy, blackhead-prone skin and acne. Its action is astringent, cleansing, detoxifying and toning. Facial steaming will be particularly beneficial.

The fragrance of juniper combines well with many

other oils, for example cedarwood, cypress, pine, lavender, geranium and citrus.

Suitable methods of use
Bathing, compresses, inhalation, massage, vaporiser/diffuser.

Precautions
Warning: To be avoided during pregnancy. May cause skin irritation in some individuals – dilute well.

LAVENDER – *Lavandula vera/Lavandula augustifolia/Lavandula officinalis*

The plant
Lavender belongs to the plant family *Lamiaceae* (*Liberate*). It originally comes from the area around the Mediterranean but is now grown worldwide. It is commercially cultivated in France, Italy, Tasmania, Great Britain and many other countries. Lavender is an evergreen shrub with aromatic leaves and flowers, and it is a great favourite in herb and scented gardens. It has a long history of use – the ancient Romans used it in bath-

ing and it has been used as a disinfectant, an antiseptic and a sedative. The dried flowers of the plant, sewn into a small pouches or bags, make delightful drawer fresheners. Lavender toilet water has been a popular product for many years.

The oil

Essential oil of lavender is obtained by steam distillation from the flowers of the plant. The oil is clear or faintly yellow and has a sweet floral odour that blends well with many other oils. Lavender is one of the most useful oils to have in the home as it is extremely safe and pleasant to use and has many functions.

The actions of lavender on the emotions are gently sedative and relaxing. It is beneficial to those whose low spirits are combined with a feeling of anxiety or vulnerability, imparting a feeling of calm while at the same time strengthening the spirits. It is a soothing addition to a massage blend and can help in the treatment of insomnia. Used in abdominal massage, lavender will help to ease flatulence and the discomfort of trapped wind in the digestive system.

The mild analgesic properties of lavender make it suitable for the treatment of headaches and muscular pain.

One of the few essential oils that can be used neat, lavender also has antiseptic properties and can be dabbed directly onto stings and insect bites and will reduce the pain of minor burns, scalds and scrapes, combating infection at the same time. In addition to this, the oil promotes healing and will help to reduce scarring.

When used in bathing, lavender oil is beneficial in the treatment of genito-urinary infections such as thrush and cystitis. In steam inhalations, it can do much to ease spasmodic coughing and will help to fight throat infections and soothe laryngitis.

Skin conditions that can be treated with lavender oil include eczema, acne, psoriasis and athlete's foot. The oil has a deodorising and antiseptic effect when used in a mouthwash.

Lavender oil is also an effective insect repellent.

Suitable methods of use
Bathing, compresses, hair care, inhalation, massage, skin care, vaporiser/diffuser.

Precautions
None. Lavender is extremely safe to use, even on babies and infants. Some aromatherapists recommend that it is

avoided in early pregnancy if there is a history of miscarriage but otherwise it is very safe for pregnant women.

LEMON – *Citrus limon*

The tree

Lemon trees are evergreen, growing to a modest height of approximately 20 feet (6 metres). The tree is native to Asia but is now grown extensively in Europe, especially around the Mediterranean. The lemon tree belongs to the family *Rutaceae*. The fruits are bright yellow in colour when ripe, and both the flowers and fruit of the tree are highly fragrant. Lemons are rich in vitamins A, B and C and have for centuries been used as ingredients in cookery. Roman women in ancient times would take a drink made with lemon juice to relieve the nausea of morning sickness in the early months of pregnancy. The flavour of the fruit is sharp and the smell is sweet and fresh. Lemon juice used to be given to sailors as a treatment for or preventative measure against scurvy and has for many years been a favourite component of homemade cold 'cures'. Lemon is an ingredient in many commercially produced sweets and other confections and is used widely by the pharmaceutical industry, the perfume industry and the cosmetics industry. Lemon is also used as a fragrance in many proprietary household cleaning agents.

The oil

Essential oil of lemon is extracted from the rind and skin of the fruit when ripe by expression. The oil is clear and has a light, fresh scent. It has a stimulating effect on the circulation and is beneficial to those who suffer from cold hands and feet and chilblains, either used in baths, footbaths or in massage blends. It has a cleansing and toning effect on the skin. The oil has antiseptic properties and is astringent, and it works well in the treatment of greasy, spot-prone skin and minor skin ailments such as boils and pimples.

In massage or inhalation, lemon oil's antiseptic properties will help combat respiratory infections such as colds, influenza, and bronchitis. In addition to this, it will also help strengthen the body's immune system.

Used in a vaporiser or spray, lemon oil is an effective insect repellent and will also help to disinfect the room of a sick person, at the same time refreshing the atmosphere and lifting the spirits.

Lemon oil is perfect for times when too many late nights and poor eating habits have given you a feeling of sluggishness or when a hard day's work or a long journey have left you feeling weary, sweaty and grubby. It is very much a 'fresh start' oil and gives an invaluable boost to the body and the morale.

Suitable methods of use
Bathing, compresses, inhalation, massage, skin care, vaporiser/diffuser.

Precautions
Lemon oil is phototoxic so should not be used prior to exposure to the sun. Apply in moderation and in low dilution as occasionally sensitisation can occur.

LEMONGRASS – *Cymbopogon citratus*

The plant
Lemongrass is a native plant of Asia, South Africa and parts of South America. It belongs to the family *Poaceae*. It is a majestic perennial grass, rapidly reaching heights of over 5 feet (1.5 metres) tall, and is

highly aromatic. Of several varieties that are cultivated, East Indian and West Indian lemongrass are the two main kinds. Lemongrass has been used as both a culinary and medicinal herb in India and Asia. Medicinal use has been mainly for the treatment of fever and infectious disease.

The smell of lemongrass is like the smell of lemons but has a harsher quality. It is very strong and is not to everyone's taste. In cookery, too, it is not universally popular – it has been said by some to taste like the smell of lemon-scented cleaning fluid!

The oil

Essential oil of lemongrass is extracted by steam distillation from the cut grass. The oil is pale yellow in colour and has an intense, lemony smell. It is used quite extensively in industry in the manufacture of various food and drink products and also in the production of household cleaners and bath and cosmetic products.

Lemongrass oil has strong antiseptic, antifungal and bactericidal qualities and can be used in the treatment of athlete's foot, thrush, and feverish infections. Used in massage, its actions are warming and stimulating, and it will help to strengthen and tone weak, tired and aching muscles. It is thus useful for athletes and for those who are recovering, but still weak from periods of illness.

Lemongrass can also benefit the digestive system. Used in massage or in inhalation it can act as an appetite stimulant and soothe an irritated or inflamed colon. The antiseptic properties of the oil will help fight gastric infections.

Like lemon oil, lemongrass oil is beneficial to oily skin and can be added to a facial steam bath to help cleanse blocked pores.

The oil is an effective insect repellent and can also be used as a general-purpose deodoriser and air freshener, either in a spray or vaporiser.

Suitable methods of use
Inhalation, massage, skin care, vaporiser/diffuser.

Precautions
Lemongrass is non toxic but can irritate broken or sensitive skin. Use carefully and in low dilution. **Warning:** Some therapists recommend that essential oil of lemongrass is avoided in early pregnancy.

LIME – *Citrus aurantifolia*

The tree

Lime trees are quite small evergreens, bearing white flowers and bright green fruit. The fruits are smaller than lemons and have a distinctive bitter taste. Limes grow in several countries and are grown commercially in Florida, Mexico, Italy and the West Indies. The tree is a member of the family *Rutaceae*.

Lime has been used quite extensively in herbal medicine for many years and shares most of the properties of lemon.

The oil

Essential oil of lime is produced by mechanical expression of the peel of the fruit. The oil is yellow/green with a strong, fresh citrus fragrance. It is used for its fragrance in the production of cosmetics, household cleaning products and perfumes. It is also used extensively by the food and drinks industries.

Therapeutically, essential oil of lime is more or less interchangeable with lemon. It is refreshing and cleansing and uplifting to the spirits. It has antiseptic properties and is astringent so can be used in the treatment of greasy and spotty skin. The bactericidal properties of the oil also make it suitable for treating skin infections such as boils.

Lime oil can also help in the treatment of respiratory complaints, such as colds and sore throats, catarrhal coughs and bronchitis.

The oil blends well with a variety of other essential oils and, used in a vaporiser or room spray, will also help to disinfect a room.

Suitable methods of use
Bathing, compresses, inhalation, massage, skin care, vaporiser/diffuser.

Precautions
Lime oil is phototoxic. After using lime oil on the skin, avoid exposure to sunlight for 24 hours. Generally nonsensitising, but may cause sensitisation in a few individuals.

MANDARIN – *Citrus nobilis/ Citrus reticulata*

The tree
Mandarin – or tangerine or satsuma, as it is now also known as, belongs to the family *Rutaceae*. The tree is

indigenous to China, in particular the southern parts, but has been grown in Europe and the United States of America for almost two hundred years. There are quite a few varieties of the fruit, which are grown commercially in Mediterranean countries and also in Brazil, the Middle East and the USA. Both the flowers and the fruit of the tree are fragrant. The fruit of the tree is sweet and appeals to most tastes. The name mandarin has its origins in times of old, when the fruit was a traditional gift to mandarins, high ranking officials, in China.

The oil

Essential oil of mandarin is obtained by mechanical expression. It is orange/amber in colour and has a pleasantly sweet citrus smell. It is widely used in the manufacture of perfumes, soaps and cosmetics and also as a flavouring agent in the food and drinks industries.

Therapeutically, mandarin is a calming oil, soothing tension and nervous irritability. It is one of the safest oils to use in aromatherapy and is thus a suitable oil for using on children, who will enjoy the scent of a bath to which mandarin oil has been added. It can help in the treatment of hyperactivity and fretfulness in children.

Mandarin oil is also valued for the beneficial effects it

has on the digestive system. Used in abdominal massage, it relieves colic, indigestion and constipation. It can be of great benefit to the elderly in this respect.

Mandarin oil is also a detoxifying agent and can help in the treatment of fluid retention.

In skin care, it is gently astringent and can benefit complexions that are prone to greasiness and/or acne.

Suitable methods of use
Bathing, compresses, inhalation, massage, skin care, vaporiser/diffuser.

Precautions
Mandarin oil is a very safe oil to use, but as there are doubts as to whether or not it is phototoxic, exposure to the sun is not recommended in the hours immediately after using the oil on the skin.

MARJORAM (SWEET) – *Origanum marjorama/ Marjorana hortensis*

The plant
Marjoram originally comes from around the Mediterran-

ean. It is an aromatic, bushy plant, growing approximately 2 feet (0.6 metres) high, with small white flowers, tinged with bluish grey. It belongs to the family *Lamiaceae* (*Labiatae*) and is a perennial. It is often confused with pot marjoram, which is a much hardier plant. The herb has a long history of both culinary and medicinal use. Its main medicinal use was for gastric complaints.

The oil

The oil of sweet marjoram is obtained from the dried flower heads and leaves of the plants by steam distillation. It is yellow-gold in colour and has a warm, spicy smell. It is used in the food and drinks industries and in the manufacture of scented bath products, cosmetics, perfumes and household cleaning products.

Marjoram oil has sedative properties and can help in the treatment of insomnia and tension. For those who are distraught with grief, 'wound up' with stress or highly emotional, marjoram can work to restore calmness of mind.

The sedative effects of marjoram mean that it is also an anaphrodisiac, that is, it reduces sexual urges.

Used in massage oil, in compresses or in baths, marjoram is valuable in the treatment of arthritis, muscular pain and swelling. It is analgesic and warming. For this reason, it can relieve dysmenorrhoea (painful menstruation). Marjoram oil is also an emmenagogue so is sometimes used in the treatment of amenorrhoea (absence of menstruation) and premenstrual tension.

In massage or in steam inhalation, marjoram oil can soothe the pain of sinusitis and headaches, including migraine.

The actions of marjoram oil on the digestive system are carminative (antiflatulence) and antispasmodic.

In massage or in bathing, marjoram oil can soothe areas of bruising and relieve the pain of chilblains.

Suitable methods of use
Bathing, compresses, inhalation, massage, vaporiser/diffuser.

Precautions
Although its sedative effects can be quite marked, marjoram is generally safe to use in appropriate dilution. **Warning:** Because of its properties as an emmenagogue, marjoram should not be used during pregnancy.

MELISSA (TRUE) – *Melissa officinalis*

The plant

Melissa officinalis, also known as lemon balm, is a fragrant-smelling herb with bright green leaves and tiny white flowers. It belongs to the family *Lamiaceae* (*Labiatae*), originally comes from the Mediterranean but is now grown extensively throughout Europe and is cultivated commercially in France, Spain and Russia. It is growing in popularity as a garden plant and culinary herb and also has a very long history of use in herbal medicine, being used to treat depression and nervous, respiratory, menstrual and digestive disorders.

The oil

The essential oil is obtained from the leaves and flowers of the plant by the process of steam distillation. The plant yields very small quantities of essential oil and therefore the oil is rather costly to produce and to buy. True melissa oil will be very expensive indeed, and it is often the case that melissa is combined with lemongrass before it is sold. The consumer must be on his or her guard, both for adulterated oil such as this and also for synthetic products.

Melissa is used for its fragrance in the manufacture of perfumed products and is also a flavouring ingredient in a variety of commercially produced food and drinks.

Therapeutically, melissa is uplifting and soothing and is useful in times of grief, trauma and associated depression. It can also be used to treat insomnia and headaches, in particular migraine.

Melissa oil can also benefit the digestive and respiratory systems. It is antispasmodic and will help in the treatment of colic and feelings of nausea. Irritating coughs and bronchitis should respond well to steam inhalation with melissa.

Suitable methods of use
Bathing, inhalation, massage, vaporiser/diffuser

Precautions
Melissa is nontoxic, but can cause sensitisation and/or skin irritation in a minority of individuals. Use well diluted.

MIMOSA – *Acacia dealbata*

The tree

Mimosa, a member of the family *Mimosaceae*, is native to Australia where it is also known as Sydney black wattle. It is a relatively small tree that has sweet-smelling yellow flowers. It has now become naturalised in several other countries in Africa and Europe. The bark of the mimosa tree is used in the tanning industry. It is also valued in herbal medicine for the treatment of diarrhoea amongst other things.

The oil

The essential oil is obtained by solvent extraction, which produces a solid concrete and a thick liquid absolute. The absolute is yellow-gold in colour and viscous. It has a woody, warm and floral scent. The properties that make mimosa beneficial for therapeutic massage are principally its soothing qualities – it has an uplifting effect on the spirits and can help those who are suffering from fear, anxiety and stress. It is mildly astringent and anti-inflammatory, and it is a valuable component in a skin-care regime, benefiting oily and sensitive skin in particular, but it is very expensive.

Mimosa is used extensively by the perfume and cosmetics industries.

Suitable methods of use
Bathing, massage, skin care, vaporiser/diffuser.

Precautions
None. Mimosa is non-toxic, non-sensitising and non-irritant.

MYRRH – *Commiphora myrrha*

The plant
Myrrh is a small shrub-like tree that grows to a height of 20–30 feet (6–9 metres). Belonging to the family *Burseraceae*, it is indigenous to Arabia, in particular Yemen, and to parts of northeast Africa, including Somalia and Ethiopia. The tree has white flowers and aromatic leaves. The trunk exudes a yellow liquid resin that hardens into solid reddish-coloured droplets. Resin collectors make incisions in the trunk of the tree to encourage it to produce larger quantities.

Myrrh, one of the gifts that the three wise men brought

from the East for the Christ child, has been used since ancient times in religious ceremonies and is an ingredient of incense. The ancient Egyptians used myrrh for embalming their dead. In herbal medicine, myrrh has a history of use as a tonic, with astringent and healing properties. It was also used as an expectorant and as a treatment for various gastric and oral problems and skin problems.

The oil

Myrrh oil is obtained by steam distillation from the resin that is exuded from the tree. It is golden to amber in colour and has a sweetish spicy, medicinal smell. It has strong antiseptic and healing properties. When used in the treatment of respiratory disorders, either in massage or in steam inhalation, its anti-inflammatory, anticatarrhal and expectorant properties can benefit coughs, bronchitis and sore throats. It can also be used in mouthwashes and gargles to treat gingivitis, mouth ulcers and oral thrush.

The effects of myrrh oil on the digestive system are stimulating. Used in massage, myrrh can help ease flatulence and stimulate appetite. It can also be used in the treatment of diarrhoea.

In skin care, either in the bath or in lotions or compresses, myrrh can be used as an antiseptic and anti-inflammatory agent. It works well on cracked and inflamed skin and can be used as a treatment for fungal infections such as athlete's foot and ringworm. In baths it can be used for the treatment of leucorrhoea and vaginal thrush. Myrrh is also thought to benefit ageing skin.

Myrrh oil is warming and relaxing and can be useful in the treatment of stress and depression. It is also used as an aid to meditation.

Myrrh oil is used in the cosmetics industry as an ingredient in soaps, cosmetics and perfumes. The pharmaceutical industry uses it in the production of oral preparations such as toothpastes and mouthwashes. It is also used in dentistry.

Suitable methods of use
Bathing, inhalation, massage, mouthwashes, skin care, vaporiser/diffuser.

Precautions
Myrrh oil is nonirritant and nontoxic when used externally. **Warning:** Do not swallow mouthwash. Not to be used in pregnancy.

MYRTLE – *Myrtus communis*

The plant

Myrtle is a large bush, growing to a height of as much as 15 feet (4.5 metres), which is native to North Africa but now growing throughout the Mediterranean area. It is an evergreen plant with shiny leaves and bright white blossom. Both leaves and flowers are fragrant. In ancient times, myrtle was sacred to the goddess Aphrodite, and it is still worn as a symbol of purity by some brides to this day. Like tea tree and eucalyptus, myrtle is a member of the plant family *Myrtaceae*. Myrtle oil is produced in several countries, including France, Morocco, Italy and Tunisia.

In traditional herbal medicine, myrtle has been used for respiratory and digestive disorders and also in skin care.

The oil

The essential oil of myrtle is obtained by steam distillation from the twigs and leaves of the plant. It is pale yellow to orange in colour and has a clean fresh smell. The oil is used in the perfume industry, particularly in the production of eau de Cologne. It is also used as a

159

flavouring ingredient in some commercially produced savoury foods.

Therapeutically, myrtle oil is used in aromatherapy for the treatment of respiratory complaints and also in skin care. Myrtle can be used to combat problem catarrh and coughing associated with this. It is also a useful treatment for sinusitis. It is bactericidal and an effective expectorant. Use in steam inhalation for best effect. The oil will also boost the immune system against colds and influenza.

In skin care, myrtle is useful for its astringent and bactericidal properties and can be used in skin preparations to treat oily skin and acne.

Myrtle has a clarifying and uplifting effect on the spirits. It can help those who are feeling low and distracted by worry.

Suitable methods of use
Bathing, inhalation, massage, skin care, vaporiser/diffuser.

Precautions
None. Myrtle is nontoxic, non-sensitising and non-irritant.

NEROLI – *Citrus aurantium var. amara* (*see also* ORANGE (BITTER) and PETITGRAIN)

The tree

Neroli, also known as orange blossom, is derived from the flowers of the bitter orange tree, also known as the Seville orange. The tree, a member of the family *Rutaceae*, is indigenous to the Far East but is now grown extensively in Mediterranean countries. The tree is a small evergreen, growing to heights of little more than 30 feet (9 metres). It has fragrant white flowers and dark orange-coloured fruits. The flowers were used traditionally in bridal bouquets as their perfume would calm the nervous bride before her wedding night. Dried flowers of bitter orange are also used in herbal medicine, taken in infusion as a tonic and blood-cleanser. Orange-flower water has been for a long time a popular aid in skin care for cleansing and toning.

Bitter oranges are used extensively in the food and drinks industry.

The oil

Neroli is named after an Italian princess who lived in

the sixteenth century and is said to have used the oil as a perfume. Neroli is an ingredient in the classic eau de Cologne and many other perfumes. The oil is obtained from the flowers by steam distillation and is pale yellow in colour with a fragrance that is fresh and floral with a hint of sharpness underneath. Although neroli is quite an expensive essential oil to buy, it is much favoured by therapists as it has many therapeutic properties and is a very safe oil to use. It is both sedative and antidepressant and is very valuable in the treatment of feelings of anxiety and nervous tension as it is calming and soothing. It is often used in the treatment of premenstrual tension, helping to balance the mood swings that are often associated with this condition. In bathing, inhalation or massage it will benefit those who have trouble sleeping, especially if the insomnia is related to distress or anxiety. It will also soothe nervous palpitations.

Neroli benefits the digestive system with its antispasmodic properties. Used in massage, in particular abdominal massage, it can help to ease colic, flatulence and stress-related colitis and diarrhoea.

In skin care, neroli is particularly beneficial to mature skins, having a rejuvenating effect. It is quite safe to use in dilution on sensitive skin and is helpful in preventing scars and stretchmarks.

Neroli combines especially well in a blend with jasmine and rose – very expensive, but quite wonderful.

Suitable methods of use

Bathing, inhalation, massage, skin care, vaporiser/diffuser.

Precautions

None. Neroli is nontoxic, non-sensitising and nonirritant. It is one of the safest oils to use in home aromatherapy.

NIAOULI – *Melaleuca viridiflora*

The tree

Niaouli is a member of the family *Myrtaceae* and is an evergreen tree with yellow flowers and very aromatic leaves. It is indigenous to Australia and some of the islands of the Pacific. Most of the oil produced commercially comes from Australia. Niaouli is still used in herbal medicine in some of the places where it grows for the treatment of respiratory disease and for antisepsis amongst other things. Niaouli is related to cajeput and tea tree and shares some of their properties.

The oil

Essential oil of niaouli is obtained from the leaves of the tree and also from young twigs by the process of steam distillation. The oil is generally colourless, or can be faintly greenish-yellow. It smells warm, sweet and quite like camphor. The essential oil is used quite extensively in the pharmaceutical industry, in particular for the manufacture of antiseptic throat and mouth preparations such as cough sweets and mouthwashes.

Niaouli has a variety of uses in aromatherapy. It can be used to treat respiratory tract infections such as sinusitis and bronchitis, especially when used in steam inhalation, and it is particularly beneficial in cases where mucus and catarrh are a problem.

Niaouli can also be used to treat various skin complaints. It is astringent and thus appropriate for the treatment of oily skin that is prone to acne. Insect bites and minor cuts, abrasions and burns can also be treated with preparations containing this essential oil, which has both antiseptic and analgesic properties.

When used in bathing or in massage (particularly massage), niaouli will bring some relief to the discomfort of rheumatism and general musculo-skeletal aches and pains. It also helps to stimulate the circulation.

Niaouli has a generally stimulating effect on the mind, clearing confusion and helping with focus and concentration.

Suitable methods of use
Bathing, inhalation, massage, skin care, vaporiser/diffuser

Precautions
Nonirritant and nontoxic. Non-sensitising. **Warning:** Avoid during the early months of pregnancy.

NUTMEG – *Myristica fragrans*

The tree
Nutmeg is native to the Middle East and the West Indies, and is cultivated in the West Indies, Indonesia and Sri Lanka. The tree is about 25 feet (7.6 metres) high and has aromatic leaves. The spice mace is obtained from the covering of the seed shell. Nutmeg is the kernel, which has been dried over heat in its shell. The spice has been used in cookery for many years. Nutmeg has been used in herbal medicine for hundreds of years, mostly for the treatment of digestive complaints, such

as flatulence, indigestion and diarrhoea, and also for kidney disorders.

The oil
Essential oil of nutmeg is obtained from the dried seeds by steam distillation. The oil is white or pale yellow in colour. It has stimulant and analgesic properties and is warming in its effect when used in massage. It is beneficial in the treatment of muscular aches and pains, rheumatism and arthritis. It can also help in the treatment of digestive problems, such as flatulence, indigestion and nausea, and can stimulate a jaded appetite. Its effects are calming and strengthening and can benefit those who are chronically tired, depressed and lacking in energy. Nutmeg oil is not recommended for home use as it can, when used in high dose, cause hallucinations and hypnosis. It is unsuitable for bathing as it is a skin irritant.

Precautions
Warning: Use only under the supervision of a trained aromatherapist. Not suitable for bathing. Avoid during pregnancy.

ORANGE (BITTER) – *Citrus aurantium var. amara* (*see also* NEROLI and PETITGRAIN)

The tree

The bitter – or Seville – orange tree is also the source of the flowers that are used to obtain neroli oil (*see* page 161). It is an evergreen, a member of the family *Rutaceae* and although native to the Far East has been growing in the countries around the Mediterranean for many years. The tree grows to a height of approximately 30 feet (9 metres). The branches have very sharp spines. The flowers of the bitter orange tree are highly fragrant. The fruit is too bitter to be enjoyable when consumed raw but is used extensively in the food and drinks industries as a flavouring ingredient and in the making of marmalade.

In herbal medicine, bitter orange peel, dried, is used in moderate quantities in treating flatulence and dyspepsia.

The oil

The oil of the bitter orange is obtained by mechanical expression of the fruit peel. It is pale orange in colour and has a fresh, rich citrus scent that is not long-lasting. In common with other citrus oils, bitter orange has a relatively poor keeping quality. Like neroli, bitter orange is soothing to the nervous system and will benefit stress- and anxiety-related problems when used in massage or in bathing. It is useful in skin care for the treatment of oily and lacklustre complexions. It is astringent, anti-inflammatory and bactericidal.

Bitter orange oil, used in massage, will have a carminative (antiflatulent) effect on the digestive system and can also help to stimulate the digestion, encourage peristalsis and ease constipation. It is also useful in the treatment of water retention and has a generally detoxifying effect.

In steam inhalation or in vaporisers, bitter orange oil has a relaxing effect while at the same time encouraging a more optimistic and cheerful outlook.

Suitable methods of use
Bathing, compresses, inhalation, massage, skin care, vaporiser/diffuser.

Precautions
Warning: Phototoxic – Avoid exposure to sunlight for twelve hours following application. Otherwise generally non sensitising and nonirritating although a very small

number of people experience some skin irritation after using the oil.

ORANGE (SWEET) – *Citrus sinensis*

The tree

A member of the family *Rutaceae*, the sweet orange is a smaller tree than the bitter orange tree and, unlike the bitter orange tree, has spineless branches. The sweet orange is native to the Far East but has been grown in Mediterranean countries, especially in Spain. It is also widely grown in Portugal and in Brazil and the United States, where it is cultivated for oil production. The flowers of the sweet orange tree are fragrant, but their scent is not as strong as bitter orange blossom. Sweet oranges are almost universally popular for their pleasant taste and are high in vitamin C. Many varieties are cultivated for consumption and for utilisation in the production of a variety of foods and drinks.

The oil

Sweet orange oil is obtained by mechanical expression of the peel of the fruit. It is light orange in colour and has a fresh, fruity smell that is sweeter in tone than that of the bitter orange. Sweet orange oil is a very safe oil to use in the home for aromatherapy and can be used on children, who generally enjoy the pleasant fragrance. Like other citrus oils, however, it has a relatively short life. Its therapeutic uses are many.

Sweet orange oil is very useful in skin care and is suitable for adding to the bath or for use in massage. It is gently astringent, conditioning and toning, and works well on all but the driest of skins, renewing a dull complexion and cleansing oily skin.

In massage or in bathing, sweet orange oil can be used with good effect as part of a programme of general detoxifying. It will also help in the treatment of fluid retention.

Sweet orange makes a pleasant and refreshing addition to room vaporisers and blends well with other citrus fragrances and also with longer-lasting fragrances such as sandalwood.

Used in massage, sweet orange also acts to the benefit of the digestive system, toning a sluggish digestion, stimulating peristalsis and gently easing problems of constipation and flatulence. It can also help combat the problems of fluid retention and mood changes that are associated with premenstrual syndrome.

In bathing, massage or inhalation, sweet orange oil will soothe away anxiety and stress and encourage a more positive and optimistic attitude.

Suitable methods of use
Bathing, compresses, inhalation, massage, skin care, vaporiser/diffuser.

Precautions
None. Sweet orange oil is very safe generally. Cases of sensitisation are extremely rare, but avoid exposure to the sun immediately after use to be on the safe side.

PALMAROSA – *Cymbopogon martinii var. martinii*

The plant
Palmarosa is a relative of lemongrass and citronella, coming from the same plant family, *Gramineae*. It is also related to gingergrass – *Cymbopogon matinii var. sofia* – which is used to obtain an oil that is similar but considered by most to be inferior in quality. The plant grows wild in India and Pakistan. It is now cultivated for commercial purposes in India and in Indonesia, the Comoros

Islands, East Africa and Brazil, all of which produce the oil. The plant has fragrant grassy leaves.

The oil

The oil is obtained from the leaves of the plant, either fresh or dried, by the process of steam distillation. It is pale yellow or green in colour and has a sweet floral smell. Palmarosa essential oil is used in the perfume industry as a fragrance ingredient. It is also used in the production of soaps and bath products.

Essential oil of palmarosa is useful in the treatment of stress-related feelings of depression. It calms troubled spirits and lifts the mood, encouraging a more optimistic view of life.

The oil can be used in the treatment of various digestive problems, combating infection and improving digestion. It can stimulate a poor appetite and can help the intestinal flora to return to a state of balance after a bout of infection or following antibiotic treatment. Use in massage or in bathing.

Palmarosa oil is very useful in skin care, where its balancing qualities make it suitable for the treatment of a variety of conditions, either associated with dry or oily skin. It helps regulate the production of sebum and also moisturises dry skin. It can be used to good effect on mature complexions, reducing wrinkles and improving the skin's tone and appearance. It will also help reduce scar tissue. Use in facial massage, creams or in facial steam baths.

Suitable methods of use
Bathing, compresses, inhalation, massage, skin care, vaporiser/diffuser.

Precautions
Palmarosa is quite safe to use in dilution. It is nontoxic, non-sensitising and nonirritant.

PARSLEY – *Petroselinum sativum*

The plant
Parsley is either grown as a biennial or a perennial, although the latter will not live for many years. It is native to the Mediterranean area, but now grows extensively throughout Europe and in parts of Asia. Parsley is a member of the plant family *Apiece* (*Umbelliferae*). In Great Britain, it is a very popular garden herb with many

culinary uses. For the purposes of oil production, it is cultivated in countries that include Germany, Holland and France.

Parsley is high in vitamins A and C. In herbal medicine, it is used for problems of the kidneys and urinary tract and also in the treatment of arthritis. Parsley is pleasant to chew on as a breath deodoriser after spicy or garlicky food. It is also a digestive aid.

The oil

Essential oil of parsley is obtained by steam distillation of the plant. Two different oils are obtained – one from the seed and one from the foliage. Parsley oil is used to treat cystitis and other urinary infections. It also acts as a diuretic. It is an emmenagogue so can be used to treat scanty and irregular menstruation.

Massage with oil of parsley can aid digestion, having a carminative and stimulating effect. Parsley oil is also used in the treatment of arthritis and rheumatism. Owing to its possible toxicity if used inappropriately, however, parsley is not recommended for use at home.

Precautions

Warning: Not recommended for home use. Parsley oil

can be toxic unless used in strict moderation. It is also a skin irritant. **Warning:** Not to be used during pregnancy. Parsley oil is an emmenagogue.

PATCHOULI – *Pogostemon cablin*

The plant

Patchouli belongs to the family *Lamiaceae* (*Labiatae*) and is tall, bushy herb with large aromatic leaves. It is native to tropical Asia. It is cultivated for commercial use in Asia, India, China and South America. The plant has white flowers and the leaves are hairy in texture. The plant has been widely used in Asia for many years as an incense ingredient. The leaves were used in woven materials to perfume them. Patchouli is also used as an insect repellent.

In herbal medicine, particularly in China and Japan, patchouli is used to treat colds, headaches and digestive upsets, including vomiting.

The oil

Essential oil of patchouli is obtained by the process of steam distillation from the leaves of the plant which are previously dried and fermented. The oil is thick and viscous and is orange-amber in colour. It has a distinctively sweet and earthy smell that is long-lasting and, unlike that of other essential oils, actually improves with age, although the fragrance of patchouli oil is not to everyone's liking – some people dislike it intensely. Patchouli oil is used in the manufacture of perfumes and soaps and is an ingredient in Indian ink.

Patchouli oil has various therapeutic applications. It is antiseptic and anti-inflammatory and can be used in skin care to treat acne, oily skin and open pores as well as minor sores that are weeping and reluctant to heal. It is also beneficial in the treatment of athlete's foot, chapped and painful skin and eczema. Patchouli is particularly beneficial to ageing skin and will also help prevent scars and stretchmarks.

When used in a massage blend, particularly in abdominal massage, or alternatively in a warm compress, patchouli can relieve constipation and combat flatulence.

In massage oil or in room vaporisers, patchouli oil is an effective room deodoriser. Used in this way, it can also be used to strengthen the spirits when exhaustion has set in and will help restore a sense of calm and determination in stressful times. The oil also has aphro-disiac properties and can benefit in particular those whose desire or sexual performance has been adversely affected by stress and fatigue.

Patchouli oil can also be used as an insect repellent.

Suitable methods of use
Bathing, compresses, inhalation, massage, skin care, vaporiser/diffuser.

Precautions
None. Patchouli oil is nontoxic, non sensitising and nonirritant.

PEPPERMINT – *Mentha piperita*

The plant
There are several different varieties of mint: peppermint and spearmint are the two that are used in aromatherapy. Peppermint is a perennial herb, a cultivated hybrid grown all over the world. It is easy to grow and spreads rapidly from underground runners. Some gardeners find this aspect of an otherwise useful herb rather irritating. The

peppermint plant is bushy, growing to approximately 3 feet (0.9 metres) in height, has soft, fragrant green leaves and small, white flowers. Peppermint belongs to the plant family *Lamiaceae* (*Labiatae*). Peppermint is grown commercially for production of its essential oils in several countries, including England, France, Italy and Russia. Peppermint is one of the oils for which an organic option is easily available.

Peppermint has a long history of use in herbal medicine. There is evidence that the herb was used by the ancient Egyptians, and in various countries it has been used as a treatment for various complaints, including indigestion, colic and flatulence, nausea (in particular during pregnancy), headaches and sore throats. The herb is often drunk in an infusion, as peppermint tea.

The oil

Essential oil of peppermint is produced by the process of steam distillation. The herb is harvested while in flower and the leaves, stems and flowers are used in the process. Peppermint oil is pale greenish-yellow and has a strong, fresh minty smell. Essential oil of peppermint is widely used as a flavouring ingredient in the food and drinks industries and by the cosmetics and pharmaceutical industries as a flavouring and/or fragrance in toothpastes, soaps, mouthwashes, bath products, perfumes and colognes.

Peppermint oil has various therapeutic uses and can be used to treat disorders of the respiratory system and the digestive tract as well as musculo-skeletal pain, in addition to being a valuable oil to use in skin care.

The anti-inflammatory and analgesic properties of the oil can benefit muscular pain and neuralgia, particularly when used in massage. Peppermint oil will also help to stimulate the circulation.

The anti-inflammatory properties of peppermint oil can also help to ease the irritation of pruritis when used in bathing. Peppermint oil is astringent and will be of particular benefit to oily skins. It is, however, irritating to some sensitive skins and should be used in dilution of no more than 1 per cent in a massage blend. Three drops are quite sufficient for bathing.

As a digestive aid, essential oil of peppermint works effectively in massage to stimulate a sluggish digestion, to relieve dyspepsia and nausea and also to ease stomach cramps and colic.

Used in steam inhalation, peppermint oil has a marked anticatarrhal and expectorant action and can do much to relieve colds and bronchitis. In a mouthwash, it can deodorise bad breath.

Peppermint oil refreshes the mind as well as the body and will help to lift the spirits, give courage and focus and clear muddled thoughts.

Suitable methods of use
Bathing, compresses, inhalation, massage, mouthwashes, skin care, vaporiser/diffuser.

Precautions
Nontoxic and generally nonirritant if used in appropriate dilution. A small chance of sensitisation in some individuals. **Warning:** Avoid during pregnancy. Do not swallow mouthwash.

PETITGRAIN – *Citrus aurantium var. amara* (*see also* NEROLI and ORANGE (BITTER))

The tree
The bitter orange tree, or Seville orange, as it is also known, is indigenous to the Far East but now grows extensively in Mediterranean countries, where it is also

produced commercially. It is an evergreen tree, a member of the plant family *Rutaceae*, with bitter tasting dark coloured oranges and fragrant blossom. Neroli is obtained from the blossom of the tree and bitter orange oil from the fruits. Petitgrain was originally obtained from the fruits when they were unripe and still very tiny, like little grains, hence the name of this oil, but is now produced from the leaves and twigs of the tree. France and Paraguay are two of the main sources of the highest quality oil.

The oil

The oil is produced from the leaves and twigs of the tree by the process of steam distillation. It is pale yellow to orange-amber in colour and smells pleasantly fresh, fruity and woody. As with neroli, bitter orange oil and also sweet orange oil, petitgrain can be used in the treatment of anxiety, stress and insomnia. It is very soothing and calming, whether used in massage, bathing or in a vaporiser.

Petitgrain works to the benefit of a sluggish digestive system, easing the discomfort of symptoms such as dyspepsia and flatulence. Petitgrain is similar in its effects to neroli and can be used as a less expensive alternative if neroli is prohibitively costly.

Like the other orange-based oils, petitgrain has a toning and astringent effect on the skin, refreshing a tired complexion and combating oiliness. It also acts as an antiperspirant.

Petitgrain is used in the cosmetic and pharmaceutical industries as a fragrance ingredient in the manufacture of various toiletries, colognes and perfumes. It is an ingredient in classic eau de Cologne.

Suitable methods of use
Bathing, compresses, inhalation, massage, skin care, vaporiser/diffuser.

Precautions
None. Petitgrain is very safe to use.

PINE, SCOTS – *Pinus sylvestris*

The tree
Pinus sylvestris, more commonly known as Scots pine, is a tall evergreen native to Britain where it was long ago the main species in the Great Forest of Caledon, covering much of Scotland. Now the Scots pine is grown worldwide and is cultivated commercially in several

countries, including Austria, the countries of Scandinavia and the United States. Scots pine belongs to the family *Pinaceae*. There are other varieties of pine that are cultivated for their oils, for example long-leaf pine and dwarf pine, but Scots pine is the one most commonly used in aromatherapy.

In herbal medicine, young pine shoots were used in bathing to treat several complaints, including rheumatism, poor circulation, skin problems and nervous fatigue. They were also used in steam inhalation for a variety of respiratory disorders. Pine was much appreciated for its insecticidal properties and was used around the house to repel parasites.

The oil

The essential oil is obtained from the needles of the tree by the process of dry distillation. It is colourless generally but can be tinged with yellow. The oil has a strong, clean, balsamic smell. The fragrance of pine oil makes it a strong favourite in the production of many soaps and other bath products. It is also used extensively as an ingredient in household cleaning products and disinfectants as well as in insect repellents.

Therapeutically, oil of pine is versatile and quite a safe

oil for home use. Its effects are refreshing and stimulating. It is particularly useful in the treatment of many respiratory ailments, such as bronchitis, influenza, coughs, colds and also asthma. It is an effective expectorant and is also antiseptic, antiviral and bactericidal. It can be used to treat respiratory tract infections either by massage or in inhalation. Steam inhalation is particularly beneficial as the steam helps to loosen excess mucus in the airways and unblock the sinuses.

Pine oil is valuable in the treatment of urinary tract infections, particularly when used in baths or sitz baths. Its antiseptic and antimicrobial properties combat infection while the patient's spirits are soothed by the refreshing fragrance.

Hot compresses of pine and massage with essential oils both work well to relieve the aches and pains of disorders such as arthritis, rheumatism and gout. Pine oil also benefits poor circulation. It is a good oil to use in the treatment of post-illness fatigue or exhaustion brought on by stress, replacing tension with relaxation and fatigue with refreshment.

Pine oil used in a room spray, vaporiser or diffuser will deodorise and disinfect the air, creating a fresh and healthy atmosphere.

Suitable methods of use

Bathing, compresses, inhalation, massage, skin care, vaporiser/diffuser.

Precautions

Pine oil is generally safe to use. It is nontoxic and generally nonirritant, provided that it is used in dilutions of less than 2 per cent. A small minority of people may become sensitised. Avoid using pine on people who already have allergic skin conditions. **Warning:** Some therapists recommend that you avoid using essential oil of pine during the first three months of pregnancy.

ROSE – CABBAGE ROSE – *Rosa centifolia*, and DAMASK ROSE – *Rosa damascena*

The plant

There are two main varieties of rose that are used for the production of essential oil for aromatherapy. *Rosa centifolia*, or cabbage rose, and *Rosa damascena*, damask rose. Cabbage rose, also known as French rose, rose de mai or rose maroc, is believed to have come originally from Persia but is now cultivated commercially, mostly in Morocco and France. The plant is approximately 8 feet (2.4 metres) in height and produces a mass of fragrant pink blooms. Damask rose, also known as Turkish rose and rose otto, is thought to be indigenous to China but is now cultivated mainly in Bulgaria and France for its oil. It is a smaller plant, which also produces abundant pink blooms. Of the two varieties, cabbage-rose oil is more widely available for aromatherapy use. Rose otto can be prohibitively expensive.

Roses were widely used medicinally in ancient times in the East for a variety of ailments, which included fever, skin problems, digestive and circulatory problems. They were also valued for their aphrodisiac properties. Symbolically, the rose signifies love and has done so for many hundreds of years. Rose hips are still valued highly for their nutritional value: they are particularly high in vitamin C.

The oil
Steam distillation of rose petals is sometimes used to produce essential oil of rose, and for many years the principal method of extraction favoured by the perfume industry was enfleurage. Essential oil of rose is extremely expensive, however, and an alternative is the absolute.

First, a concrete is obtained through solvent extraction of the rose petals and then, once the solvent has been removed, the absolute is separated from the concrete using alcohol.

The essential oils of both cabbage rose and damask rose are yellow in colour, while the absolutes are deeper in hue, being orange-red. The absolute is almost solid at room temperature, becoming liquid when the bottle is held and gently warmed in the hand. Both essential oil and absolute have a rich, deep, sweet floral smell. Beware of imitations: synthetic copies of rose oil abound and it is also quite frequently adulterated before being sold.

Rose oil is extensively used in the perfume industry. Being an ingredient of more than a third of the fragrances. It is also used in the manufacture of toiletries and cosmetics and sometimes as a flavouring agent. Rose water – a by-product of the steam distillation process – is used in cookery and for cosmetic purposes.

Rose oil is a pleasant and safe oil to use in aromatherapy and is suitable for a variety of uses. It is expensive, but its strength ensures that one or two drops added to a blend will transform it. Cabbage-rose oil and damask-rose oil have similar properties and effects.

Rose oil relaxes and strengthens, imparting a feeling of calm and wellbeing. It is beneficial to use in times of stress and will bring relief to many stress-related conditions, soothing frustration and irritability and lifting the spirits. It can be used to good effect on children and is enjoyed by most people in massage blends or in bathing. Rose oil is also delightful to blend with other essential oils in a vaporiser.

In the treatment of gynaecological problems, rose oil can be particularly beneficial. It is useful in the treatment of premenstrual tension and in menopausal difficulties such as heavy menstrual bleeding. Its effects are balancing, and it can also help to regulate infrequent or scanty menstruation. Like jasmine, rose oil has aphrodisiac qualities and can benefit both sexes by increasing libido.

Rose oil can also benefit the respiratory system and can be used to treat coughs and allergy-related respiratory complaints.

The effects of rose oil on the digestive system are detoxifying, anti-inflammatory and strengthening. It can be used to treat constipation and nausea and is also thought to have a tonic effect on the liver and gall bladder.

Rose oil is an extremely valuable oil for skin care. It is

anti-inflammatory and soothing, which makes it suitable for the treatment of dry and itchy skin, and it will also help to tone a tired complexion. It is suitable for use on sensitive and ageing skin.

Rose oil also has a beneficial effect on the circulation.

It is important to point out that although rose oil is very costly, a little of this intoxicating fragrance goes a long way in a blend.

Suitable methods of use
Bathing, inhalation, massage, skin care, vaporiser/diffuser.

Precautions
Safe to use; nontoxic, nonirritating and non-sensitising.
Warning: Use of rose oil during early pregnancy is not advisable unless under the supervision of a trained aromatherapist.

ROSEMARY – *Rosmarinus officinalis*

The plant
Rosemary, symbol of remembrance, originally comes

from the Mediterranean area but is now grown worldwide and is cultivated for oil production in France, Spain and Tunisia. Rosemary is a member of the plant family *Lamiaceae* (*Labiatae*). It is a relatively easy herb to grow and is popular as a flavouring ingredient in the cookery of many countries. It is also a favourite in scented gardens and herb gardens. Planted alongside a path, where the leaves will give off their delicious fragrance every time someone brushes past the plant, rosemary is a delight to grow. The herb grows as a small bushy shrub with grey-green aromatic leaves, like needles, all along the stem. The flowers of the plant are small and pale greyish blue in colour. Rosemary has been used in herbal medicine for centuries and also had considerable religious and spiritual significance in some countries. It was believed in several cultures to give protection against evil spirits. In medieval times it was used as a fumigating agent against the plague. The herb has been used to treat respiratory, digestive, skin and nervous complaints and is still recommended as a general stimulant. Rosemary was also used as a treatment for depression and general debility. The stimulating effects of the herb on the mind and body have long been appreciated.

The oil

Essential oil of rosemary can be extracted from the whole plant by steam distillation, but a better quality oil is obtained if only the young leaves and flowering tips are used. The oil is either pale yellow or colourless and has a fragrance that is strong, fresh and herbal. The fragrance of the oil does not, however, closely resemble that of the plant itself. Rosemary oil is used extensively in the perfume and cosmetics industries, in the manufacture of soaps, shampoos and other toiletries and in perfumes and colognes. It is also used in the production of many food and drink products.

The effects of essential oil of rosemary are warming, stimulating, strengthening and toning, both on the body and the mind. It is thus a good all-round tonic oil to use and has many therapeutic applications.

Rosemary has particular benefits for the circulatory system. Used in a bath or in massage it will stimulate a poor circulation and relieve the discomfort of cold extremities.

Rosemary oil can be used to good effect in bathing, massage or adding fragrance to a room to stimulate the mind, helping concentration, improving memory and relieving mental fatigue: 'Rosemary for remembrance'.

(It is interesting to note that the ancient Greeks wore sprigs or garlands of rosemary at times when they wanted to achieve this effect.)

Rosemary is a good oil to use in massage or bathing both before and after strenuous exercise. It is therefore invaluable to have in the house if there are athletes, walkers or cyclists in the family. It will help to tone the muscles and help prevent against strain before exercise. Following exercise, it will soothe aches, pains and stiffness. Rheumatism and arthritis can also be relieved by using rosemary oil, which is soothing and warming either in massage and bathing or with the use of compresses applied to the affected areas of the body.

The pain-relieving properties of essential oil of rosemary also make it useful in the treatment of headaches, and its stimulating properties help to restore concentration and revitalise the spirits, particularly when fatigue from overwork has set in.

The stimulating effects of rosemary will work for the benefit of the digestive system, and it can be used to treat flatulence, colic and an irritated colon. Abdominal massage can be particularly beneficial. Massage with rosemary oil also has a detoxifying effect on the body, stimulating lymphatic drainage.

Rosemary oil is antiseptic and antimicrobial and can be used in the treatment of colds, influenza and bronchitis. Use in steam inhalation or, for a comforting warming effect all over, in bathing or massage. It can also be used in a mouthwash to combat oral and throat infections. When used as a room fragrance, rosemary gives off a delicious aroma while at the same time disinfecting the atmosphere.

Rosemary oil is a popular oil to use in hair care. It can be applied in a massage blend rubbed into the scalp and can be used to treat hair lice and scabies. It also counteracts greasy hair, seborrhoea and dandruff and it may also be of benefit in some cases of hair loss (alopecia).

In skin care, rosemary oil is particularly beneficial for oily skins that are prone to spots as it is antiseptic and astringent.

Suitable methods of use
Bathing, compresses, hair care, inhalation, massage, mouthwash, skin care, vaporiser/diffuser.

Precautions
In the correct dilution, rosemary oil is generally safe to use. **Warning:** Should be avoided during pregnancy. Not

suitable for use by sufferers of epilepsy or high blood pressure.

ROSEWOOD – *Aniba rosaedora*

NOTE
Rosewood has been harvested for years without any programme for replacing the trees with new plantings. This has been very damaging environmentally. Rosewood is slow-growing and resources are becoming increasingly limited. The rainforests have suffered greatly as a consequence of the felling of the trees for timber and oil. Those who have any regard for the environment will probably choose not to use this oil, in spite of its therapeutic benefits, unless given proven assurance that the oil comes from a sustainable source. Many (and most reputable) suppliers of essential oils will also refuse to sell the oil unless it meets environmentally conscious criteria.

The tree
The tree is a tropical evergreen of medium size and grows in the Amazon basin. It is a member of the family *Lauraceae*. The timber has been used for many years

in the production of high-quality furniture and is also exported to Japan for the manufacture of chopsticks. Peru and Brazil are the largest producers of rosewood oil.

The oil

The essential oil of rosewood is obtained from wood chippings by the process of steam distillation. The oil is colourless or pale yellow and has a sweet, pleasantly woody fragrance. Rosewood oil was formerly used as a source of linalol for the perfume industry, but now most linalol is synthetic. Rosewood oil is still used in the manufacture of perfumes and perfumed products and is also extensively used in the food and drinks industries.

Therapeutically, rosewood is balancing, calming, uplifting and toning. It is a sensual oil to use in massage or in a vaporiser to scent a room, and it blends well with a variety of different oils, in particular the citrus and floral oils. It can help to relieve tense headaches, soothe stress and aid concentration.

Rosewood oil is antiseptic and antimicrobial, and it strengthens the body's immune response. It can be used in massage, bathing or inhalation to help combat influenza and similar infections. It has reasonably good expectorant properties and can help to soothe dry coughs. Not only will rosewood oil help the body to fight off troublesome infections, it will also make sufferers feel better in themselves and can help combat the depressive symptoms that are often associated with a severe bout of influenza.

In skin care, rosewood oil can be used for a variety of purposes. It is anti-inflammatory and will soothe dry, sore complexions. It is widely appreciated for treating ageing skins, scarring, dermatitis and eczema.

Suitable methods of use
Bathing, compresses, inhalation, massage, skin care, vaporiser/diffuser.

Precautions
None. Rosewood oil is nontoxic, non-sensitising and nonirritant.

SANDALWOOD – *Santalum album*

The tree
Sandalwood, a member of the family *Santalaceae*, is native to India where it is now cultivated for commercial

purposes, particularly in the southern state of Karuataka, formerly known as Mysore. The sandalwood tree is a small evergreen, a parasite that gets nutrients from photosynthesis but draws the water and minerals that it requires from the roots of a host tree. (Mistletoe belongs to the same family.)

There has been some concern over depleting resources in recent years, but this problem is now being resolved with replanting programmes that have been initiated by the Indian government, which also regulates the quality of the oil that is produced. Another variety of sandalwood, Australian sandalwood, is also used for essential oil production but the Indian sandalwood is considered superior and is thus the one of choice.

Sandalwood has been used for its perfume for some four thousand years in the East. In powdered form it is burned as incense and it has been used as a component in the embalming process. Its ceremonial and religious uses include weddings, funerals and festivals. It was also used therapeutically in Eastern traditional medicine for fighting off disease.

The wood was used for building and for ornamental carvings, in particular for temples.

The oil

Sandalwood oil is obtained from the heartwood of the tree, which has previously been dried and powdered, by steam distillation. It is used as a perfume and a fragrance fixative in cosmetics, aftershaves, colognes and perfumes. It is one of the essential oils that appeals equally to both sexes. Sandalwood oil is a component of many varieties of incense. It also has value as a flavouring in some commercially produced food and drinks.

Sandalwood oil is safe to use in massage, bathing, skin care and inhalation. It will do much to relieve anxious feelings of depression. It has a relaxing, soothing effect on the spirits. It is cooling, quietening and calming and is often used by those who meditate. Sandalwood oil can help break the vicious circle of insomnia, wherein the sufferer has trouble sleeping, becomes anxious about not sleeping and then finds it even harder to sleep because of the anxiety. Sandalwood will induce a state of relaxation that is conducive to sounder, easier sleep.

The skin can benefit from the use of sandalwood oil as an emollient and anti-inflammatory agent on dry, cracked and tender skin. It cleanses and softens and is pleasant to apply in dilution to the face after shaving. It is also mildly astringent. Its fragrance has an almost universal appeal. Sandalwood is also valued for its aphrodisiac properties and is believed to increase sexual enjoyment, in particular for men.

Used in the bath, sandalwood oil is extremely beneficial to the genito-urinary system and can help in the treatment of vaginitis, leucorrhoea, cystitis and urethritis. It is anti-inflammatory and antiseptic and can also be used to treat some sexually transmitted diseases.

Used in steam inhalation, sandalwood can help in the treatment of dry coughs and heavy, mucousy colds. It is an effective decongestant and can help to clear catarrh.

Suitable methods of use
Bathing, compresses, inhalation, massage, skin care, vaporiser/diffuser.

Precautions
None. Sandalwood oil is nontoxic, non-sensitising and nonirritant.

STAR ANISE – *Illicium verum*

The tree

Native to southeast China, the tree is a medium-sized evergreen, growing up to 40 feet (12 metres) in height. The fruits are star-shaped, with between five and thirteen seed pockets radiating from the centre. The tree, a member of the *Illiciaceae* family, also grows in India and Japan. The main source of the fruits and oil is China although some star anise is exported from India as well.

Star anise has a long history of use in traditional Chinese medicine, where it has been used as a digestive aid, an antispasmodic and for the treatment of coughs for thousands of years.

The oil

The essential oil of star anise is produced from the fruits by steam distillation. The oil is clear or tinged with yellow and smells very sweet, rather like liquorice. It is effective at masking other less pleasant tastes and smells and is used extensively by the pharmaceutical industry as a flavouring ingredient, especially to render certain medications more palatable. It is also used as a fragrance ingredient in various toiletries and as a flavouring in the manufacture of a number of foods and beverages.

Therapeutically, star anise is a sedative oil and is valued for its soothing, relaxing properties. It is a useful oil to use in massage or vaporisers to achieve a comforting sense of calm.

Star anise is particularly beneficial to the digestive system, for the relief of distressing symptoms such as hiccups, flatulence, stomach cramping, colic and indigestion. It can be used in massage blends for this purpose and massaged gently over the stomach and abdomen.

In steam inhalation, star anise oil is an effective expectorant so helps clear excess mucus from the airways. and also does much to soothe coughs and colds.

In general massage or in compresses the oil will relieve muscle cramping and can also be used to treat joint and muscle stiffness and aches and pains.

Star anise has very similar properties to the oil that is distilled from the herb aniseed, but as aniseed is a dermal irritant and not recommended for home use, star anise is a safer alternative, provided that it is well diluted. It is not recommended, however, for bathing.

Precautions

Warning: Use star anise well diluted (2 per cent dilution or less) and in moderation as it can have a narcotic effect. Star anise oil an cause irritation in some individuals with damaged or very sensitive skin. Otherwise, it is nonirritant if used in appropriate dilution and is safer to use than aniseed, from which a similar essential oil is extracted.

TARRAGON – *Artemisia dracunculus*

The plant

Tarragon is a perennial herb native to Europe, Siberia and Mongolia. It is now grown all over the world and is a popular culinary herb, particularly in France, which is one of the main sources of the essential oil. Other producers include Holland and the United States of America. The name *dracunculus* means 'little dragon' and in France, tarragon is known as *herbe au dragon*, or the 'dragon herb'. It is a member of the family *Asteraceae* (*Compositae*).

Tarragon grows well in sunny situations but can be damaged by frosts in winter. It grows to a height of approximately 2 feet (0.6 metres) and the slender aromatic leaves are dark green in colour. The flowers are small and yellow. Two varieties are cultivated: Russian and French.

In ancient times, the herb was used as an antidote for various poisonous animal and insect bites. The root of the plant was also used to treat toothache. In Persia, tarragon was eaten to stimulate the appetite.

The oil

Essential oil of tarragon is obtained by the process of steam distillation from the leaves of the plant. The oil is either colourless or pale yellow in appearance. It has a strong, spicy smell, fresh and green in quality. It is used for its fragrance in the manufacture of toiletries and perfumes, and for its flavour it is extensively used by the food and drinks manufacturing industries.

Therapeutically, tarragon has a stimulating effect on the digestion. It is also antispasmodic and can relieve hiccups, flatulence and colic. Tarragon has therapeutic value in the treatment of some menstrual dysfunctions. The effects of the oil on the circulation is stimulating. However, tarragon oil has a degree of toxicity and is not recommended for home use.

Precautions

Warning: Not suitable for home use. Avoid during pregnancy.

TEA TREE – *Melaleuca alternifolia*

The tree

Tea tree grows as a shrub or small tree in Australia. It is a member of the family *Myrtaceae*. Its leaves are slender, like needles, and the flowers are either yellow or purple in colour.

The leaves of the tree have a very long history of use by the aboriginal people of Australia, who used them to make an infusion for drinking – hence the name 'tea tree'. The leaves were also used, crushed, for application to wounds and sores. The properties for which the tree has been appreciated for many hundreds of years make the essential oil of tea tree one of the most exciting and versatile oils in aromatherapy.

The oil

Tea-tree oil is extracted from the leaves of the tree by steam distillation. It is pale yellow-green in colour and has a strong, spicy and pleasant odour reminiscent of camphor. It is used very extensively in the pharmaceutical and cosmetics industries in the manufacture of antiseptic and germicidal preparations, gargles, toothpastes, bath products and skin treatments. Organically produced tea-tree oil is now widely available.

Tea-tree oil is one of the most useful oils in aroma-therapy – many would claim it is the most useful. It is safe to use, it can be applied neat to the skin, and it has powerful antiseptic, disinfectant, antiviral, antifungal and bactericidal properties, which make it of value in the treatment of a wide variety of ailments. It also stimulates the body's immune response against infection. Tea-tree oil is a 'must' for the first aid kit.

The immuno-stimulant, antiviral and bactericidal prop-erties of tea-tree oil make it particularly beneficial in the treatment of colds and influenza and other respiratory tract infections. For this purpose, steam inhalation is rec-ommended. Alternatively, use the oil in a massage blend. For throat infections and painful mouth infections, for example oral thrush, gingivitis and ulcers, tea-tree oil can be used in mouthwashes and gargles. It is also ef-fective in combating bad breath and can be used to treat cold sores.

For treating genito-urinary infections, such as cystitis, thrush, herpes, pruritis and urethritis, tea-tree oil can be used in a bath, or a sitz bath. It is very soothing and will combat infection.

In the area of skin care, tea-tree oil can be used to good effect for the treatment of a wide variety of problems. It can be used in facial steam treatments, lotions and massage blends for the skin. It can be dabbed neat onto spots and blemishes, insect bites, minor burns and stings. It is antiseptic and will also bring relief from discomfort. It can be used to treat fungal skin infections such as athlete's foot and ringworm. Leg wounds and ulcers that are difficult to heal, particularly if the sufferer is elderly and has poor circulation, can benefit from treatment with tea-tree oil in a bland carrier such as almond oil.

Research continues into the therapeutic applications of tea-tree oil and there is optimism that there are still further benefits to be derived from its immunostimulant and antimicrobial properties.

Suitable methods of use
Bathing, compresses, inhalation, massage, mouthwashes, skin care, vaporiser/diffuser. Can be applied neat to the skin.

Precautions

Tea-tree oil is nontoxic and nonirritant. There is a small chance of sensitisation in a few individuals, but this is rare.

THYME, COMMON – *Thymus vulgaris*

The plant

Common thyme is a member of the plant family *Lamiaceae* (*Labiateae*). There are many varieties of thyme. Common thyme is derived from wild thyme. It is native to, and grows extensively in, the area around, the Mediterranean. The plant is low-growing and shrub-like with small white or pale blue/purple flowers and has aromatic leaves. It also grows in other European countries and in North Africa, and it is popular in many countries as a culinary herb.

The herb has been used therapeutically since ancient times. The Greeks burnt it to fumigate buildings against infectious disease. It was also a symbol of courage to the ancient Greeks. The ancient Egyptians used thyme in the process of embalming. The Romans used it to flavour cheese.

In herbal medicine, thyme is used in combination with

other herbs for the treatment of various gastric and respiratory ailments and for fever.

The oil

Two different oils are produced from the herb. The first is red thyme oil, which is obtained by steam distillation from the leaves and flowers of the plant. The second, white thyme oil, is produced after a second distillation process has been carried out. Red thyme oil, as its name suggests, is brownish red in colour. It has a strong, spicy, warm smell. White thyme oil is very pale yellow in colour and smells sweeter and less pungent than red thyme oil. Red thyme oil is much stronger and more of an irritant than white thyme oil; the latter, therefore, is safer to use.

Thyme oil is used extensively in the pharmaceutical industry, in the manufacture of antiseptic mouthwashes, toothpastes, throat lozenges, disinfectants, etc. The cosmetics industry uses it as a fragrance ingredient in soaps, shampoos and bath products.

Thyme oil is a powerful antiseptic and germicide. It also has a stimulating effect on the nervous system. It can, however, irritate the skin and should only be used well diluted. In bathing, a dilution of only 1 per cent is recommended.

Thyme oil can be used to treat respiratory infections such as colds, influenza and bronchitis, either in steam inhalation or in massage. It also has beneficial effects on the respiratory system if used in a vaporiser. It is an expectorant so also helps relieve spasmodic coughing. An added benefit of thyme oil is its immunostimulant properties, which help the body to fight off infection. Used in a vaporiser, diffuser or room spray with other antiseptic oils it will help to disinfect the atmosphere in a sick-room.

Thyme oil can be used to treat a variety of infections of the genito-urinary tract, including cystitis and urethritis.

Used in massage in particular, thyme oil can bring relief from the symptoms of arthritis and rheumatism and will also combat the stiffness and aches that are associated with overexertion and sports-related muscle strain. It also benefits the circulatory system with its stimulating effects and can combat low blood pressure.

Provided that it is well diluted, thyme oil can be used in skin care for a variety of purposes. It can benefit oily skin and acne and has been shown to be effective against lice and scabies.

The effects of thyme oil on the nervous system are

stimulating: combating mental fatigue, nervous debility and symptoms of stress such as headaches.

Suitable methods of use
Bathing, compresses, inhalation, massage, vaporiser/diffuser

Precautions
Use with care. Dilute well. Do not use on broken or sensitive skin. **Warning:** Not suitable for children, epileptics or those who are prone to high blood pressure. Avoid the use of thyme oil in pregnancy.

VETIVER – *Vetiveria zizanoides*

The plant
Vetiver is a grass, a member of the family *Poaceae* (*Gramineae*) and it is native to southern India, Sri Lanka and Indonesia. It grows to a height of approximately 6 feet (1.8 metres). It has deep, strong roots and is planted in some countries to protect the soil from erosion. It is now cultivated in several countries, including India, Reunion, Java, Haiti and Brazil.

Vetiver roots have been used for hundreds of years for their fragrance and the grass is used for weaving mats.

The oil

The essential oil of vetiver is produced from the roots by steam distillation. Vetiver oil is used extensively in the perfume industry and in the manufacture of scented toiletries. It also has uses in the food industry. The essential oil is reddish dark brown and has a woody, earthy smell that is almost musty. It is quite viscous and benefits from being gently warmed in the bottle before it is used, to make it flow more freely. The oil has a strong odour (that may not be to everyone's taste) and should be well diluted to avoid it being too overpowering in a blend.

Therapeutically, vetiver oil has a profoundly relaxing effect on the nervous system, relieving tension and stress. It can be used to good effect in the treatment of insomnia. In India, vetiver oil is known as 'the oil of tranquillity'.

In baths or in massage, vetiver is beneficial in the treatment of the symptoms of disorders such as arthritis, rheumatism and aching, stiff muscles. It is warming and comforting and will help to relieve the tension that is often associated with chronic pain.

Vetiver oil also benefits the circulatory system, stimulating and warming, especially when used in combination with massage.

In skin care, the antiseptic and slightly astringent properties of vetiver can be used to good effect in the treatment of oily skin that is prone to spots.

Suitable methods of use
Bathing, compresses, inhalation, massage, skin care, va-
poriser/diffuser.

Precautions
None. Vetiver is nontoxic, non-sensitising and nonirritant.

YLANG YLANG – *Canaga odorata var. genuina*

The tree
Ylang ylang is indigenous to Indonesia, the Philippines,
Java and Madagascar. Madagascar is one of the main
sources of the essential oil, which is also produced in
Reunion and the Comoro islands. The tree grows to a
height of approximately 65 feet (19.8 metres), and it is
from the large yellow or pink fragrant flowers of the

tree that the oil is extracted. The yellow flowers are considered superior to the pink ones for purposes of oil extraction.

The flowers have a long history of use in skin care and in the prevention of infection. The aphrodisiac properties of the flower have been appreciated for many hundreds of years, and in Indonesia ylang ylang blooms were traditionally scattered on the beds of newly-wed couples on their wedding night.

The oil

The flowers are steam distilled to produce the essential oil. A total of four distillations take place. The product of the first distillation is known as ylang ylang extra and is the most expensive and the highest quality. The three following distillates, known as grades I, II and III, are progressively diminished in complexity and quality. Ylang ylang oil was an ingredient of macassar oil, which was very popular in Victorian times as a treatment for the scalp, stimulating hair growth. The oil is pale yellow and has a powerful sweet, floral fragrance that has a hint of spiciness. It is similar in many respects to jasmine oil.

Ylang ylang oil is used extensively in the perfume industry and also in the manufacture of cosmetics, soaps and toiletries. Ylang ylang extra is the oil sought after for high quality perfume production.

Ylang ylang has many uses in aromatherapy. It has a sedative effect on the nervous system and will calm anxiety and help with problems of insomnia. It will help relieve feelings of depression, especially if these are stress induced. Because of the strength of the fragrance, which can become overpowering and in some cases can cause headaches and/or nausea, ylang ylang is best used well diluted.

In bathing, room perfuming or in massage, particularly in sensual massage, the aphrodisiac properties of the oil can be used to good effect, encouraging relaxation and enjoyment.

Ylang ylang also benefits the circulatory system and can calm palpitations and help to lower raised blood pressure. It will also help to treat hyperpnoea (excessive breathing after exercise).

In skin care, ylang ylang can soothe insect bites and will have a balancing effect on the skin, making it beneficial in the treatment of acne and oily skin as well as dry skin.

Suitable methods of use
Bathing, massage, skin care, vaporiser/diffuser.

birth. Whilst much of the literature is very useful, anyone who is embarking upon the great adventure of pregnancy, whether for the first time or not, would be well advised to consult a professional aromatherapist for additional personal advice. Every person and every pregnancy is different. You stand to gain greater benefit and more reassurance from taking individual advice from an expert. Both you and your baby deserve it.

Aromatherapy and Children

Babies

Babies are highly responsive to touch and to smell from the moment of birth onwards, and there is a great deal of benefit to be derived, both for the mother and for the child, from the use of massage and aromatic oils.

Very new babies should not be treated with essential oils but can be massaged gently with almond oil or olive oil. Make sure the baby is warm and comfortable before you start, and stroke the child's body and limbs gently and rhythmically. If the baby seems unduly fretful then discontinue the process. It is unlikely to be the massage that is causing the child's distress, but little is to be gained from persisting if the child is unable to relax because of discomfort or hunger.

Once the baby is four weeks old, you can start to introduce essential oils and use them twice or three times a week. Chamomile and lavender are quite safe to use in the appropriate dilution: at this stage, use one drop of essential oil to one tablespoonful of carrier oil, no more. Take great care to keep the oil away from the baby's face. After a few months you can introduce other oils: mandarin, neroli and rose are generally considered suitable.

You can also place a bowl of hot water with a couple of drops of essential oil in the baby's room: mandarin or lavender will be particularly soothing and fragrant. If the child has a cold, you can put a drop of eucalyptus oil in a bowl of hot water close to the cot to help clear a snuffly nose.

As is the case with pregnancy, you will be able to find a great deal of literature on the subject, but for both your and the baby's benefit and for your own peace of mind, your first step should be to consult a professional.

Young children

A wider variety of oils may be used on children as they grow older. Never use oils that are known to be possible skin irritants on children, however. From when the baby is one year old onwards, you can use two drops of essential oil per tablespoon of carrier. From when the child reaches the age of around six or seven years, you can use half the quantity of essential oil that you would for an adult. Normal adult doses can be used after the age of twelve or thirteen.

Massage

There are several forms of therapy that make use of different forms of massage: reflexology, shiatsu, Swedish massage, physiotherapy and sports treatments to name a few. Aromatherapy makes extensive use of massage in treatment, and aromatherapists study the specific techniques involved in detail, along with anatomy and physiology, when they are training.

Physiotherapy and sports medicine

Massage in physiotherapy and in sports medicine tends to concentrate on specific areas of the body where there is muscle strain or injury. It tends to be used as a localised treatment for a localised effect, being its aim remedial rather than relaxing. It is therapeutic, like aromatherapy massage, but unlike aromatherapy massage it is used for treating a part of a person rather than a whole being. Neuromuscular massage, a technique that uses relatively heavy pressure compared to other forms of massage, is used with other techniques in sports therapy. Mechanical devices may also be used in sports massage. Therapeutic massage of this sort is best left in the hands of those who have been specifically trained.

Swedish massage

Swedish massage, which dates from the nineteenth century, is widely used by the beauty industry and uses techniques of kneading, rolling and squeezing the flesh and effleurage (*see* Massage Techniques page 230). It is a relaxing form of massage and helps to improve the circulation and boost lymphatic drainage. Aromatherapy massage is not quite the same as Swedish massage, but employs some of the same techniques. Swedish massage is quite safe and the techniques involved can be used, if desired, in the application of essential oils at home.

Reflexology

Reflexology is gaining popularity once more in modern times, but it is an art with ancient origins, coming from the East. Reflexology works on the principle that specific zones of the body can be treated with massage of corresponding areas – reflexes – elsewhere. The foot is most commonly used for treatment, certain spots on the foot being selected for particular attention to treat corresponding areas elsewhere in the body. Reflexology, practised professionally, is not only used for treatment but also for diagnosis. Thus non-specific pain in the body that is of uncertain origin can be pinpointed quite precisely by the reflexologist upon examination and massage of the patient's foot. Reflexology is thought to be particularly beneficial in the treatment of endocrine disorders and for general stimulation of immunity and lymphatic drainage.

Shiatsu

Shiatsu, like reflexology, comes from the East. It is an ancient art that works along principles that are very similar to those of acupuncture. Thus it concentrates on the meridians along which the body's energy flows. These meridians must remain clear for the body to function properly. Like acupuncture, shiatsu concentrates on specific points on the body where pressure is applied, but unlike acupuncture, which is very precise and requires years of learning, elements of shiatsu can be practised by people who have a much more basic knowledge than that of the acupuncturist. Shiatsu massage is quite firm and the pressure can be painful at times. It can be given as either as a localised treatment or as a whole-body massage, working along the energy meridians from head to foot.

Aromatherapy massage

Aromatherapy massage has something in common with each of the above. Although it is the usual practice for an aromatherapist to give whole-body massage, it will often be the case that specific areas of the body are given particular attention if required. For example, aching muscles in the back or tension in the shoulders and neck can be given specific treatment during the course of the massage procedure. At home, if free time is limited and a full-body massage is out of the question at any particular moment, great benefit can still be gained from more localised massage to 'problem' areas. A soothing abdominal massage using appropriate oils can do much to help when digestion is sluggish or when periods are painful. A shoulder and neck massage will smooth out knots of tension and help to relax the subject. If a whole-body massage is not convenient or practicable, then a careful foot massage will benefit not only the feet but the whole person. The principles of reflexology and aromatherapy are quite compatible and indeed many aromatherapists use reflexology in the treatment of their patients. The added bonus of reflexology is that foot massage can quite easily be carried out by individuals on themselves. There are many helpful books on the topic for those who are interested.

A variety of techniques will be used by the professional aromatherapist. As in Swedish massage, kneading and effleurage will be used quite extensively, but in addition to this some deep pressure can be employed, for example in the specific area of muscle pain, and attention will be paid to the meridians of the body to allow energy to flow freely and help the body to restore harmony within itself. The massage will be 'tailored' to the individual's needs, just as much as the choice of the oils that are used. Whether the overall effect of the massage is stimulating, relaxing or balancing will depend upon what is required.

Those who have visited a professional aromatherapist will attest to the fact that they feel quite different when the treatment is finished. The oils generally take around twenty to thirty minutes to take effect so their benefits will already be being felt by the time the massage is complete, and the effect of the oils, combined with massage, can be quite astonishing. Those who are visiting an aromatherapist for the first time may be advised to leave the car at home: a deeply relaxing massage can make the subject very sleepy.

Aromatherapy massage at home

Precautions

Massage is generally quite safe, but there are certain circumstances that render it inadvisable. Massage is inappropriate (and can sometimes be dangerous) if any of the following conditions are present:

  epilepsy
  coronary disease
  fractures, open wounds, severe bruising, haemorrhage
     (or history of same), recent scarring
  fever, or infectious disease with fluctuating temperature
  contagious skin disease
  sunburned skin
  osteoporosis
  high blood pressure
  varicose veins
  areas of acute inflammation
  nausea
  undiagnosed swellings or lumps

Preparation

The first thing to ensure is that you are fit to carry out

the massage. If you are suffering from back pain you cannot massage properly and you risk further injury to yourself. Similarly, it is best to massage a partner, friend or family member only if you yourself feel that you have the energy. Choose a time when you feel calm and relaxed but not tired. Ensure that you are wearing comfortable, light, loose clothing that will not hinder your movements or make you become overheated. Avoid long, wide sleeves – short sleeves are preferable – and don't wear necklaces or pendants that could dangle over the subject and cause irritation. For the same reason, if you have long hair, keep it tied back out of the way. Wash your hands thoroughly and make sure that your nails are clean and short. Before beginning massage, make sure that your hands are warm.

Ensure that the room is very warm. Lighting should be good but not too bright. Massage can be carried out on the floor, with something soft laid down for the subject to lie on, but it is easier for the person carrying out the massage if a surface such as a long table (not too high) can be used. Beds are generally unsuitable – the massage surface needs to be firm – but a thin, firm mattress placed on the floor or table will make your subject more comfortable and thus make it easier for both of you to achieve maximum benefit. Have all the oils that you might require ready to hand, and some tissues to wipe your hands on or to wipe up any accidental spillages. Soft music can be played in the background if so desired to provide additional enjoyment and a calm, soothing atmosphere. Ensure that you will not be interrupted by telephones or other people. If there are others in the house, ask them to stay out of the room and to try to keep noise down to a minimum. The latter two aims can be particularly hard to achieve when there are children in the house. Waiting until they are asleep or choosing a time when they are out of the house might be preferable.

Talk to your subject for a while to find out how he or she is feeling mentally and physically in order to allow you to prepare a massage blend that is most suitable for the moment. Make sure that at least one hour has passed since your subject's last meal. Remember that if you are new to aromatherapy, it is best to keep your blends simple. As you prepare your blend and mix it with your carrier oil, ask your subject to undress and lie on the table or floor. Cover your subject with towels and ensure, during the course of the massage, that you keep him or her covered, apart from the area on which you are working.

Massage techniques

Effleurage

Effleurage is widely used in massage and is quite a simple movement to carry out. Effleurage is basically a form of stroking, varying the pressure to suit, using the whole hand. Using effleurage on the back is a good way to commence a massage as it relaxes the subject and spreads the essential oils over a large surface of skin right from the start. Thus, as you work on other areas of the body, the oils will already have penetrated the skin and started to work. Begin gently, working towards the heart all the time to promote venous return. Keep the strokes smooth and continuous. Pressure can be reasonably firm but should not be heavy.

Petrissage and kneading

These two techniques are quite similar, petrissage being suitable for areas where there is not much flesh, i.e., when the bone is close to the skin, whereas kneading is used on fleshier areas of the body such as the thighs or upper arms. Use fingertips and the balls of the thumbs for petrissage, moving small areas of skin round between them in circular direction, clockwise with the right hand, anticlockwise with the left. The hands do not slide over the flesh as in effleurage; rather the flesh is moved, one small area at a time, by the fingers and thumbs.

Kneading is carried out with straight fingers and thumbs lifting an area of flesh and passing it to the other hand. Pressure can be quite firm but should not be painful.

Petrissage and kneading help to break down deposits in the tissues and stimulate circulation and lymphatic drainage, helping the body to rid itself of toxins.

Abdominal massage
Abdominal massage can be used to treat a variety of gynaecological and digestive complaints. Heavy pressure should never be used and particular care should be taken if the subject is pregnant or menstruating. Use gentle effleurage, working in a clockwise motion round the abdomen.

Back massage
When massaging the back, it is best to start with effleurage, working with one hand on either side of the spine. Work from the bottom of the spine upwards, stroking upwards and, as you reach the shoulders, outwards. The subject should find this wonderfully relaxing. This is a particularly pleasant way to spread the oil from your hands

onto the patient's skin. Keeping your hands on the subject, continue round over the shoulders and down the sides of the subject towards the waist. While pressure need not be very firm, it should not be too soft as the subject might find an over-gentle touch tickly.

Working on more specific areas of the back, kneading can be used on the fleshier areas at the sides. Keep your movements smooth and flowing. As one hand leaves the subject's body, the other should remain in contact, giving the patient (remember, he or she will be face down and unable to see what you are doing) a sense of security. Work up either side of the spine using petrissage, making small, circular movements with your thumbs as you move upwards from the lumbar region towards the neck. Keep the pressure firm without being heavy-handed. You should be able to feel the subject's back relax as you do this, and any tenseness you may have noticed in the way he or she has been lying on the table should visibly reduce. As you become more practised at massage, you will be able to detect specific little knots of tension in the muscles as you work, and you can give them specific attention as required.

Menstrual pain can be treated with massage of the lower back. Use petrissage, starting at either side of the sacrum (the base of the spine above the coccyx or tail bone) and working your way outwards towards the sides of the hips. Keep your movements slow, using fairly firm pressure and moving your thumbs in fairly wide circles. Keep the rhythm of your movements steady and soothing.

Finish off a back massage as you started, with effleurage over the whole area. Leave the subject to rest for a few moments before rising.

Neck and shoulder massage
This can be done as part of a whole-body massage but can also be carried out when time and facilities do not permit the full treatment. It is a wonderful tension and stress reliever and can help in the treatment of tension headaches. The subject need not be lying down; he or she can sit on a chair, facing backwards, with the arms folded on the back of the chair supporting the head. A pillow placed under the arms can make this position more comfortable. If preferred, the subject can sit on a chair leaning over a table, provided that the table is high enough to avoid back strain.

Use effleurage initially, stroking in an anticlockwise direction, working round from shoulders to neck. Use petrissage on the neck at each side of the spine, working your way from the base of the neck upwards to loosen knots of tension. With the flat of your hands over the top of the subject's shoulders, work your thumbs round in circles around the fleshier area at the top of the shoulders, pushing more firmly with upwards movements of the thumbs. Finish the shoulder massage with effleurage.

Foot massage

As has already been mentioned, foot massage can be used to benefit the whole body. Foot massage has the added benefit of being an easy way to self-help in aromatherapy. Treat yourself to a warming footbath to which aromatic oils have been added, then settle down in a comfortable position in a warm room and give yourself a foot massage.

When giving a foot massage to someone else, ensure that both of you are in a comfortable position. You will probably find that unless the subject is lying on the floor or on a couch, it is best if you sit in chairs facing each other. The subject places his or her foot on a stool or low table (use something to pad the surface) immediately in front of you. It is better if your seat is slightly lower than the subject's seat.

Work all over the foot, from toe to heel with small circular movements of your fingers and thumbs. Pay particular attention to areas of discomfort or pain – these are signs of problems elsewhere in the body.

A thorough general foot massage will undoubtedly be beneficial, but further benefit will be gained if you apply the principles of reflexology. There are many helpful books on the subject. The best way to learn is through practice, so find a book with a clear, easy-to-read chart of the reflexes on the feet and prop it up within clear sight as you massage. Initially, you may find that referring to the chart does interrupt the 'flow' of the massage somewhat, but further practice sessions will help to familiarise you with the reflexes. In time, you will be able to dispense with the chart and concentrate totally on the real foot in your hands.

Leg massage

Leg massage can be wonderfully relaxing for tired and aching muscles and is extremely beneficial for stimulating a sluggish circulation. **Warning:** Varicose veins, however, should never be massaged. If you are going to carry out a leg massage, begin with the feet (*see* above), then work your way up to the legs. Start with effleurage movements, stroking firmly upwards from foot to hip. Knead the fleshier areas of the legs, working first on the calves and then the thighs. Grip the subject's calf with your thumbs at either side of the shin and your palms, one immediately above the other, over the calf muscle, pulling gently but firmly outwards, round and back. For the thighs, work up and round with straight fingers and thumbs, moving the flesh from hand to hand, always keeping contact with the skin.

Face massage

Face massage should always be gentle. Cover the subject's eyes with cotton pads before commencing. Using gentle effleurage, stroke from the centre of the face outwards. Start beneath the chin, working out towards the ears, then from the centre of the face across the nose, up and out towards the temples. Stroke from the centre of the forehead out towards the temples. Press more firmly at the sides of the temples and work your fingertips round in circles to ease away tension.

To improve circulation, softly tap your fingers over the subject's face, again working from the centre outwards.

Finish off the facial massage with effleurage.

Home Selection:
Preferred Essentials

As you become familiar with different oils and more expert at blending them for personal use, you will, needless to say, build up your own stock for use in the home. There are some oils, however, which are particularly useful to have in the house at all times.

Citronella
Citronella has many therapeutic applications and its deodorising and insect-repellent properties make it particularly useful to have in the house.

Eucalyptus
Eucalyptus oil is an essential standby, especially in the winter when coughs and colds lurk everywhere, waiting to strike. It can be used in a vaporiser, both to treat respiratory infections and to disinfect the room. It is a valuable oil to use in steam inhalations for respiratory problems and it will also do much to ease stiffness in muscles and joints when used in massage.

Grapefruit

Fresh and fragrant, grapefruit oil is energising and detoxifying and particularly useful for times when tiredness and
overindulgence strike and you are feeling bloated and
sluggish. If you need a fresh start, you need grapefruit oil.

Jasmine/ylang ylang

Jasmine oil is very expensive, so if you find the price
prohibitive, you may prefer to use ylang ylang. These
two oils have been chosen for inclusion in the list of preferred essentials primarily for their luxurious, sensual,
feel-good qualities. We all deserve something like this
from time to time.

Lavender

Lavender oil is invaluable. As first aid for burns and
stings and for the treatment of a variety of skin problems
it is extremely useful to have in the house. It is also
soothing and calming and makes a relaxing and
pleasingly scented addition to massage or bath blends.
It also can be used to treat several respiratory and
digestive ailments.

Mandarin

If you have children, mandarin oil is a useful essential oil to keep in stock. Its soothing, calming properties will come in useful when they are fretful and 'overwound' and its pleasantly fruity fragrance is almost universally popular. If you don't have children, it is still worth keeping in store for your own benefit. We all get overwound sometimes, after all.

Rosemary

Rosemary oil is a wonderful tonic for the body and the mind. Keep it in the house for use in baths and massage blends to relieve muscle and joint stiffness, soothe headaches, banish mental fatigue and boost flagging spirits. It can also be used in skin care and in the treatment of respiratory complaints.

Tea tree

Like lavender oil, tea tree is a first-class first aid oil to have in the house. Its antiviral, antibacterial and fungicidal properties make it suitable for the treatment of a wide variety of complaints, particularly of the skin, the respiratory system and the genito-urinary system.

Warning

The following essential oils should *never* be used under any circumstances as they are extremely poisonous.

bitter almond	sassafras
boldo leaf	savin
calamus	southernwood
horseradish	tansy
jaborandi leaf	thuja
mugwort	wintergreen
mustard	wormwood
pennyroyal	wormseed
rue	yellow camphor